Current Issues
in Nursing

DATE DUE

	DATE DUE	
NOV 17 2003		

Current Issues in Nursing

EDITED BY

MOYA JOLLEY

Lecturer, Institute of Advanced Nursing Education
The Royal College of Nursing

AND

PETA ALLAN

Director for Professional Standards
and Development
United Kingdom Central Council for Nursing
Midwifery and Health Visiting

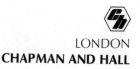

LONDON
CHAPMAN AND HALL

First published in 1989 by
Chapman and Hall Ltd
11 New Fetter Lane, London EC4P 4EE

© 1989 Chapman and Hall

Typeset in Times 10/12pt by
Leaper & Gard Ltd, Bristol

Printed in Great Britain by
St Edmundsbury Press Ltd
Bury St Edmunds, Suffolk

ISBN 0 412 32850 X

British Library Cataloguing in Publication Data

Current issues in nursing.
    1. Medicine. Nursing
    I. Jolley, Moya II. Allan, Peta
    610.73
    ISBN 0-412-32850-X

Contents

Contributors

Peta Allan, MA, DipFEd, SRN, ONC, RNT, FBIM
   Director for Professional Standards and Development
   United Kingdom Central Council for Nursing, Midwifery
   and Health Visiting.

Trevor Clay, MPhil, RGN, RMN, FRCN
   General Secretary
   Royal College of Nursing, London

Claire Goodman, MSc, BSc, NDN, RGN
   Lecturer in Nursing Research
   Dept. of Nursing Studies
   King's College
   University of London

Christine Hancock, BSc(Econ), RGN
   General Manager
   Waltham Forest Health Authority
   General Secretary Designate, Royal College of Nursing, London
*Moya Jolley, MA(Ed), BSc(Econ), DipEd, SRN, RNT, Dip in
Nursing Education (Lond)*
   Lecturer, Institute of Advanced Nursing Education
   Royal College of Nursing, London

Audrey Miller, MSc(Nursing), BA, SRN, RMN, RNT
   Lecturer, Dept. of Nursing Studies
   University of Wales College of Medicine

Colin Ralph, MPhil, RGN, Dip in Nursing (Lond)
   Registrar and Chief Executive
   United Kingdom Central Council for Nursing, Midwifery
   and Health Visiting.

Jane Robinson, PhD, MA, AIPM, RGN, ONC, RHV, HVT, Cert Ed
   Director, Nursing Policy Studies Centre
   University of Warwick

Acknowledgements

The editors wish to extend their grateful thanks to all the contributors to this book. Without their enthusiasm and hard work this book would not have been possible. Thanks go also to Miss Maude Storey for writing the Foreword.

Appreciation and thanks are also extended to Miss Helen Thomas, Assistant Librarian in the Library of Nursing at the Royal College of Nursing, for her untiring efforts in checking and preparing references; and to Mrs Jean Smith for all her help and support in preparing the final typescript.

Preface

The editors' intention in the production of this book was to provide a realistic picture of the present state of nursing. This has been presented from a number of different but inter-linked perspectives. The decades since the inception of the National Health Service have been ones of significant change, both in society at large and in the field of health care. The period has witnessed political, economic, social, scientific and technological change taking place ever more rapidly; whilst, in terms of health care, demand and expectations continue to increase apace. Nursing, throughout the period, has been influenced by, and has responded to, these prevailing influences, and continues to do so.

Contributors to this volume have sought to examine in depth some of the current issues in nursing at the present time. Each chapter examines a specific issue in the current nursing context and is, therefore, capable of standing alone. But considered together the chapters enable many aspects of the current debate on, and development of, nursing to be seen as a whole.

It is hoped that this book will serve two fundamental purposes. First, to stimulate debate and activity by all nurses in their particular sphere of influence, and in the wider world of nursing. Second, it aims to inform those undertaking pre- or post-registration nursing programmes and thus assist their understanding of the state of nursing.

The editors' purpose in presenting this book is to assist nurses to maximize their contributions to the factors which lead to improved standards of patient and client care.

Foreword

MAUDE STOREY

President,
Royal College of Nursing

The growth and development in and around nursing and the complexity of nursing has never been so marked as at this time. Many of the major developments require informed comment as an aid to understanding. A book which will bring into focus some of the major areas of professional development, highlighting current and future issues, is a valuable resource to assist in providing an important knowledge base.

This is an historical period in the life of the nursing profession. I write this foreword at a time when we have received positive announcements on two long sought developments on clinical career grading systems and on a reform of nurse education. Each of these achievements will have effects not only upon individual career progression and on the education of nurses, but upon the future development of nursing in its widest sense: the skill mix in providing care, the standard of care given, development of primary health care and in many different areas which as yet many of us can scarcely envisage.

In a large gathering of nurses, following the Secretary of State's announcement of an agreement to the fundamental principles enshrined within 'Project 2000', a member of that group exhorted those present to await judgement until *they* have written the 'fine print'. Here was evidence of a great lack of understanding, for in truth the nursing profession must recognize that it is nurses not 'they', whoever 'they' may be, who are now responsible for writing the 'fine print' and developing the means whereby reform can be achieved.

Nursing has traditionally been seen as an art and a science. However, with a nursing education system which, in the past, has created the artificial separation between the practical and theoretical elements, we have hardly reinforced the art and science base.

There is still much more that needs to be done to ensure that the art of nursing is comprised of sane nursing actions informed by sound knowledge and research. Nurses need to gain insight about the developing state of the art, should know how far education, the linkage of theory to practice and research in nursing has progressed. More importantly, that knowledge should inform on how much further these matters need to be developed in the pursuit of excellence in care provision.

Most nurses work within the NHS and thus the importance of an understanding of the context in which practice takes place for the majority of the profession is vital. This subject quite rightly holds an important place in this book. Any developments in nursing are greatly influenced by the context in which nursing is performed.

The working through of the, as yet, uneasy relationship between functional management of nursing and general management has and continues to present a challenge. Never has there been a greater need for sound leadership, for the recognition of potential leaders and for their development.

Some leaders within the profession have, for many years, recognized that developments in nursing which have the greatest professional impact depend, for achievement, upon fighting within the political arena. Great professional desires, such as those specified earlier, could only have been achieved in that scenario which for many nurses is as yet unknown and fearful territory to tread.

Dame Sheila Quinn in her address to an RCN Congress exhorted nurses to 'get political – stay professional'. That is still an important axiom. Nurses must recognize the importance and reality of politics in every aspect of life, not least nursing. There is a need to educate, to overcome our political naïveté, to begin to feel more comfortable and sure in the political sphere and above all, to rid ourselves of remnants of antagonism which still exist on the matter of further involvement. Without political acumen the future of nursing will continually be decided by others outside the profession and by those who have learnt to play the political game.

Nursing, in its professional emergence, must depart once and for all from the dependence upon others to dictate its practice. In recent years great stress has been laid upon the nurse's individual professional responsibility and accountability for nursing actions.

The word 'autonomy' rather than 'dependency' has been emphasized. These are the inevitable steps in the development of a
profession and its practitioners. The greatest professional maturity
is reached, however, when the profession accepts its responsibilities, its accountability and its autonomy in the actual practice of
nursing, is comfortable with the concepts and gains from these the
confidence to recognize that nursing can only truly survive and be
effective in a collegiate type of interdependence with other health
care workers. Such maturity ensures that the interdependent provision of health care is not seen as a threat to nursing. Health care
provision requires a sharing of practice if total health care for individuals, families and communities is to be achieved.

This book cannot, and does not, attempt to address all the
major issues in nursing development but rather emphasizes some
of the vital ones. It will assist the understanding of some of the current
matters facing the profession; how the present state was reached
and, hopefully, will stimulate questions, comment and debate as to
where future initiatives should and will take the profession.

1 The professionalization of nursing: the uncertain path

No-one has ever done anything great or useful
by listening to voices from without.
Florence Nightingale (1860)

It could be said that the twentieth century is the century that witnessed the rise of the professions and professionals. Great varieties of occupations now seek to be considered professions, from engineers to architects, hairdressers to footballers and tennis players. All seek the recognition, social prestige, and economic rewards believed to be concomitant with the status of a profession, and seen as accruing certainly to the older established professions such as law and medicine.

At first this professionalization was viewed in positive terms, as being highly functional for society. Professionals were seen as working to, and maintaining high standards, as being client rather than reward orientated, and as acting as guardians of the individual and public interest. These functions still constitute the main difference, theoretically, between a profession and a non-profession.

Nursing, as an occupation, has not stood aloof from this trend, and even a brief review of the literature on professionalism and professionalization seems to indicate that nursing has devoted an inordinate amount of attention to the subject and that it has generated, and continues to generate, some degree of controversy among nursing writers, both in Great Britain and in the United States at the present time.

Cynics might suggest that only those who are unsure regarding their status and membership of a profession use the term with any great frequency. A possible reason therefore that so much ink has been spilt on the subject resides in the fact that nursing has not yet fully attained professional status, though it has traditionally been accorded the courtesy title of profession from very early days. Some modern writers prefer to categorize it as an emergent or semi-profession (Etzioni, 1969) (see Table 1.1).

In order to pursue the subject further it is necessary to define the concepts of 'profession' and 'professionalization' and to examine briefly the ways in which sociologists and others have sought to clarify and analyse the many facets of this somewhat complex subject area.

Immediately problems arise as lack of clarity and precision of definition pervade much of the literature. Millerson (1964b) suggests this is due to a lack of consensus among sociological writers concerning the traits to be emphasized in theorizing.

Prior to the 1960s sociologists tended to emphasize the positive functions and achievements for the established professions. Earlier writers, as Freidson notes, focused on the analysis of professional norms, role relations, and interactions in the work setting (Freidson, 1983). Later, post-1960s writers have become increasingly critical, examining the relationship of professions to political and economic élites, and to the State. Others have considered the subject in relation to the class system and to the market.

Dingwall and Lewis (1983) defined certain professionals as '. . . honoured servants of the public need . . . distinguished by their orientation to serving the needs of the public through the schooled application of their usually esoteric knowledge and complex skill'.

The concept of 'profession' cannot be defined in terms of any one particular characteristic. Two broad types of approach have generally been adopted by sociologists when writing on the subject: the 'trait' approach and the 'functionalist' approach.

The trait model consists of lists of 'attributes', whereas the functionalist models are mainly concerned with elements seen to have functional relevance, either within the professional/client relationship, or for society as a whole.

Many writers, adopting the trait approach, have attempted to draw up lists of so-called attributes of a profession. One of the earliest writers in this field was Abraham Flexner. His criteria are still referred to by modern writers, and it may therefore be helpful to enumerate his suggested attributes here.

According to Flexner (1915) a profession is

1. basically intellectual, carrying with it high responsibility;
2. learned in nature, because it is based on a body of knowledge;
3. practical rather than theoretical;
4. in possession of a technique that can be taught through educational discipline;
5. well organized internally;
6. motivated by altruism.

Carr-Saunders and Wilson (1933) in their study, some twenty years later, defined a profession as 'an occupation based upon specialised intellectual study and training, the purpose of which is to supply skilled service or advice to others for a definite fee'. They went on to enumerate a number of factors characterizing a profession, including possession of authority, a code of ethics, community sanction, and existence of a professional culture among their list of attributes, but laid particular emphasis on the importance of a systematic body of knowledge. Those disciplines requiring rigorous and lengthy study of such a complex body of knowledge were ranked as professions, while those requiring less were ranked as near professions.

This emphasis on possession of a body of knowledge as a dominant characteristic of a profession is supported by more recent studies, such as that by Becker, who defined professions as 'occupations which possess a monopoly of some esoteric and difficult body of knowledge . . .' (Becker, 1962). Other writers have considered other characteristics such as autonomy, to distinguish a profession from other occupations (Freidson, 1983).

The trait approach, however, is viewed by some sociological writers to be inadequate. It rarely considers the social conditions in which professionalization takes place, particularly the prior existence of other powerful occupational groups, or the influence of governments to impose their definition on the organization and practice of an occupation. A later chapter in this book will examine in depth the influence of politics in, and on nursing as an occupation. Potential clientele may also influence the policy. practice and direction of professional development. Another criticism of the trait model lies in the fact that it is based on the seemingly uncritical acceptance by sociologists of what professionals have said about themselves.

Wilensky (1964), taking a developmental approach, viewed occupations as progressing through five stages in their passage towards becoming professions. The initial stage consisted of an occupational group emerging, engaging in full-time, mainly non-manual activity. This would be followed by the establishment of training and selection procedures for entrants to the occupation; the formation of a professional association, an elaboration of a code of ethics, and the achievement of public recognition, together with political agitation to achieve legal protection, and support to control entry and modes of practice. The foregoing is really a description of areas in which an emerging profession must participate in its transactions with other occupations in society, though the sequence may be both time and context bound.

Flexner, mentioned earlier, took learning and intellectual endeavour to be the most important of all criteria when considering professions. 'Professions are, as a matter of history – and rightly so, "learned professions"; there are no unlearned professions; unlearned professions – a contradiction in terms – would be vocations, callings, or occupations.' (Flexner, 1915.)

Larson (1977) saw professions as being established on three dimensions: first, the cognitive, relating to knowledge and techniques; second, the normative, relating to service and ethics; and third, the evaluative, relating to autonomy and prestige.

Goode (1969) suggested that professions possessed two core characteristics: those of prolonged training and service orientation.

Table 1.1 demonstrates the characteristics of professions as seen by a selected number of writers. As can be seen, opinions vary and some might be tempted to agree with Millerson's comment that 'of the dozens of writers on this subject few seem to agree on the real determinants of professional status' (Millerson, 1964a). Opponents of the trait approach suggest that the model engenders a rigid view of what a profession actually is and fails to lay sufficient emphasis on the dynamic processes involved.

The increase in professionalization is viewed by many writers as being a characteristic feature of the occupational structure of advanced industrial society. Vollmer and Mills (1966) see it as a process that may affect any occupation to a greater or lesser

Table 1.1 Characteristics of professions according to selected authors

Characteristics

	Flexner	Carr-Saunders and Wilson	Cogan	Habenstein	Barber	Freidson	Moore	Larson	Greenwood	Goode	Hughes	Schein	Becker	Kornhauser
Knowledge	X	X	X	X			X	X	X			X	X	X
Theoretical base	X								X					
Altruism	X				X	X								
Code of ethics	X				X	X			X					
Autonomy							X	X				X		X
Service					X	X				X				
Competence				X										
Commitment														X
Professional association	X				X				X		X			
Prestige				X							X	X		
Authority							X			X				
Trustworthiness							X	X						

From Moloney (1986)

extent. Like many other processes it does not occur in a vacuum and therefore cannot be fully comprehended without a consideration of certain other aspects of the society in which it takes place. Vollmer and Mills also make the point that increasing professionalization can be both an antecedent and a consequence of significant social change.

Johnson (1972) considers how the term 'professionalization' can be used in a variety of ways. First, it may be used to refer to broad changes in occupational structure whereby professional jobs increase numerically in relation to other occupations. Second, it may be used in a way implying an increase in the number of occupational associations attempting to regularize recruitment and practice in a specific occupation. The term may also be utilized to describe a more complex process whereby an occupation comes to exhibit attributes essentially professional in nature; or refer to a process whereby an occupation passes through predictable stages of organized change, the end-state of which is professionalism.

Theodore Caplow (1954) has enumerated five steps in the process of professionalization:

1. the establishment of a professional association,
2. a change of name, reducing identification with a previous lower status,
3. formation of a code of ethics,
4. political agitation,
5. establishment of training facilities and minimum qualifications.

Larson (1977) viewed professionalization as

> the process by which producers of special services seek to constitute and control a market for their expertise. Marketable expertise is a crucial element in the structure of inequality, therefore professionalisation appears also as a collective assertion of special social status, and as a collective process of upward social mobility.

The writer goes on to comment that it is an attempt to translate one order of scarce resources – special knowledge and skills – into another, social and economic rewards.

Professionalization viewed in these terms can be seen as clearly linked to both the economic and the class systems of society. In addition to these factors the influence of gender roles is also of significance. Vollmer and Mills (1966) state that 'the most highly professionalized occupations have been, historically, almost the exclusive province of men'. Female-dominated professions have been consistently retarded in terms of professionalization. Many possible reasons are advanced in explanation of this situation, including perceived lack of female commitment in career terms, and the powerful influence of stereotypical thinking, summed up in the belief that 'a woman's place is in the home'.

In considering the processes of professionalization it should be borne in mind that most, if not all, professions depend to a certain extent on large-scale organizations and on the State. This must inevitably mean bureaucratization to a greater or lesser extent.

The role of the professional within a bureaucracy has been a focus of interest for many sociological investigators over the past two decades. Particular areas for potential conflict and tension have been isolated. Long ago Emile Durkheim, whilst viewing bureaucratic structure as essential to industrial society, was also aware of its dangers in terms of its potential to stifle spontaneity, initiative and creativity, whilst being also dysfunctional in terms of its lack of flexibility, developing 'trained incapacity' at an individual level, and allowing for rules to become no longer a means to an end, but an end in themselves. Later writers' findings confirm rather than dispute Durkheim's comments.

It may not be surprising therefore, bearing in mind the above factors, that modern writers tend to see the areas of conflict for a professional within a bureaucratic setting as relating to the following:

1. resistance by the professional to bureaucratic rules,
2. rejection of bureaucratic standards where these conflict with professional ones,
3. resistance to bureaucratic supervision,
4. conditional loyalty only to the bureaucratic organization concerned.

A later chapter in this book examining the National Health Service in depth will consider some of these problems in further detail, as will the chapter dealing with issues in nursing management.

It should be remembered that the concept of profession and the process of professionalization are not viewed in positive terms by all observers and analysts of the social scene. One writer refers to professionalism as the ideology of the few who hold power (Heraud, 1973) and it has recently been criticized in terms of its legitimation of inequality.

Freidson comments that:

> economists have been inclined to note the closed, monopolistic character of the professionalized labour market, while political scientists have been inclined to concern about professions as privileged private governments. Policy makers have been inclined to see professional experts as over-narrow and insular in their vision of what is good for the public.

One of the severest critics of professionalism among modern writers is Ivan Illich (1977) who comments 'in any area where human need can be imagined these new professions, dominant, authoritative, monopolistic, legalised and, at the same time, debilitating and effectively disabling the individual – have become exclusive experts of the public good'. He goes on to suggest that 'they are more entrenched and international than a world church, more stable than any labour union, endowed with wider competence than any shaman, and equipped with a tighter hold over those they claim as victims than any mafia'.

Illich's view may be thought to be extreme by some, but he is not alone in his criticism of the modern growth of professions, and the role of the professional, particularly in relation to the so-called 'caring professions', where the processes of professionalization are seen to be potentially inimical to the caring role. O'Brien (1978) warns that 'full professional recognition would undoubtedly enhance the social and economic standing of nurses, but it would not necessarily improve patient care'.

It would appear therefore that the concepts of profession, professionalism and professionalization are surrounded to some extent by conflicting views and controversy. Problems of definition and differing views regarding dominant characteristics remain, whilst criticism of the role of professions in society continues to be heard.

Nursing would do well perhaps to heed the points made by Johnson (1972) that an occupation must be clear about what a claim to professional status entails, what is actually being aimed for, what the consequences of such claims will be, and under what conditions they are likely to be successful.

Moloney (1986) suggests that nurses may sometimes use the term profession, or professionalism, without always being aware of its depth of meaning or the problems involved in achieving it. She goes on to comment that professionalism is not about high pay and increased status, but about controlling nursing practice and having autonomy. Some nurses, she observes, appear unwilling to assume responsibility and fail to demonstrate commitment to professional development. Professionalization requires a degree of role change and constitutes a cost in terms of time, energy and resources. Even so they remain terms that are frequently used in nursing debate, and written about often at considerable length.

A decade ago Johnson (1978) commented that nursing 'had long attracted the title of "profession" and its members have bathed in the reflected glory of professional status without possessing a number of the features essential to the establishment of that status'. Gamer (1979) comments that the title has been held, as mentioned earlier, from courtesy, but suggests that few could claim full professional status for nursing at the present time, though asserting the potential for it. She sees the idea of professionalism as the most important and powerful in the whole belief system of nursing.

A modern British writer considers that nursing has now become obsessed with the idea of professionalism and that the preoccupation with professional status has now ousted the idea of nursing as a vocation, which is now being seen as out-dated (Salvage, 1985).

In this process British nursing would seem to be following a direction similar to that recently outlined by Margaret Parsons (1986), writing of the North American context, where she suggests that there has been a transition in American nursing from self-confidence to obsessive self-scrutiny. She comments that in accepting other professions as its standard, nursing has thereby deprived itself of its own unique identity. She goes on to suggest that nursing stands today in great need of the advice of its founder not to listen to 'voices from without'. Nursing has become vulnerable due to its own internal struggles and has fallen prey to sociologists who propose a single route to occupational credibility. Although Parsons was writing specifically of the American context parallels can be drawn with the British situation and the warnings noted.

Hall (1980) states that the

> primary responsibility of nursing, and therefore the purpose of professionalism is to provide care direct to the patient, client, family or community; it is concerned with maintaining, promoting and protecting health, treating the sick, and providing rehabilitation. It deals with the psychosomatic and psycho-social (and spiritual) aspects of life as these affect health, illness and dying.

No doubt this is true, though the ideal and the real need to be carefully sifted. The use of the term 'professional' is value-laden, suggesting behaviour which is, in some way, more skilled, dedicated and autonomous, and generally of a higher standard. This may not always be so and there are many who would challenge that view.

As mentioned earlier, the professions have been under attack from many outside them, who tend to view them as élitist, status-seeking groups, in the state of becoming monopolistic oligarchies. Both medicine and law tend to demonstrate some of the more negative features of professions. Social scientists cite restricted entry and monopoly of service as examples. Both these arise, it is argued, not out of concern for public welfare, but in self-interest and material gain. It has been suggested that the future presented by professionalism is not necessarily all that nurses would desire.

It would appear that aspiring to professional status has both negative as well as positive implications. Goode (1969) warns of these extreme outcomes of the professionalization process to be avoided by emergent professions. First, achieving cohesion and using the new-found strength this may impart merely to improve incomes, with little concern about the ideal of service. Second, as the knowledge base of the occupation grows, splits into subgroups may occur potentiating future disunity. Third, where an occupation is, or can be, supervised by a bureaucracy, and the substance of its work requires little autonomy, there is the danger of absorption into the higher levels of bureaucratic positions. All these outcomes undermine the claim to the trust and autonomy of professionalism.

Katz (1969) suggests that nurses are under pressure from their leaders to become professional while doubting their ability to do so; a doubt shared by many of their medical colleagues. In his study he drew attention to many problems encountered by nurses in the hospital context, including the fact that the nurse 'has no clearly formulated body of professional knowledge that is recognized and accepted by others'. He pointed also to the considerable antagonism existing between physicians who wanted dependable, servile nurses, and nurses themselves who wanted professional dignity and autonomy. Two things were seen to be needed for development towards professional status; the growth of a body of knowledge, and a change to a relation of colleagueship with physicians. It is interesting to note that although two decades have elapsed the findings of the study are not yet out of date, and the problems not yet satisfactorily resolved. Katz, as is well known, was writing of the American nursing context, but many of his points also have relevance for the British context.

There are indeed many difficulties for nursing as an occupation in seeking professional status. One of these is weight of numbers. Professions, as stated earlier, are élites. With truth White (1982) comments that '500,000 nurses will never become an élite'. Another difficulty which commentators on the nursing scene often allude to is the problem of disunity and the fact that nursing, as an occupation, may to its detriment speak with more than one voice.

Habenstein and Christ (1955) in the United States, identify three groups within nursing: the professionalizers, the traditionalizers and the utilizers. These differing groups do not necessarily share the same aspirations. The professionalizers, it is suggested, focus less on the patient and more on the importance of knowledge and skills, whereas the traditionalizers are viewed as lacking in intellectual focus, though dedicated and uncritical in terms of hospital practices. The utilizers appear not to be committed to professional knowledge or hospital tradition, wishing to be judged only on efficacy and diligence in task performance.

White (1984) in Great Britain, has also drawn attention to differing groups within nursing (though using different nomenclature), having differing philosophies and differing aspirations. She suggests that the greatest barrier to professionalization of nursing is the attempt to achieve professional status for all nurses, commenting that many do not want it if it is to be bought by educational means.

Bevis (1982) draws attention to four philosophical systems arising within the historical setting of nursing, which Clay (1987) in a more recent study suggests are all currently present in nursing and contribute to the lack of purpose to effect change. These systems Bevis (1982) refers to as asceticism, romanticism, pragmatism and humanism, each placing different emphases on aspects of nursing values, beliefs, approaches to and behaviour within a nursing context. Contrasting groups in these terms within an occupation would seem inevitably to present problems of disunity and uncertainty.

In considering the professionalization of nursing it would be an omission to exclude a brief consideration of the influence of the feminist movement. Feminism, according to Chinn and Wheeler (1985) is 'a world view that values women and that confronts systematic injustices based on gender'. Feminist writers argue that women occupy an oppressed position in society resulting from patriarchal dominance. Many also point to the far-reaching effects of socialization and the educational processes to which women are exposed, where a powerful bias favouring the male is believed to exist. Pinch draws attention to the fact that theories of developmental psychology, including moral development, takes the male as their model for the mature adult, and fail to legitimate women's experiences (Pinch, 1981).

Both Ashley (1972) and Melosh (1982), in their separate studies, make the point that failure to achieve professional status is in part due to the fact that approximately 97% of nurses are women, a fact which in itself precludes them from such a goal. Speedy (1987), in a recent article comments that

> the dual identity of 'woman' and 'professional' creates a dilemma because there is a contradiction between the characteristics and behaviour associated with the female sex role and those required for professional achievement. In general the socialisation of women is associated with renunciation of achievement and autonomy, and acceptance of nurturing, complying and dependent roles.

Florence Nightingale's view that a good nurse was a good woman, and the suggestion by Pinch that the prototype for professional nursing evolved from the mother's role in the family and her duties in situations of illness, injury and death, support the above statement. Oakley (1984) suggests that the view of the good nurse as a good woman can be considered as both the strength and the weakness of nursing as a profession, particularly in relation to altruism. Altruism may be seen, not only as an aspect of both being a woman and being a nurse, but also as a social strength. The community benefits from altruistic service but the individual often fails to. White (1984) comments that 'whilst altruism is an ideology shared by all nurses we must understand that it is not the route to professionalism'.

Maresh (1986) suggests four barriers to professionalization: feminization, by which is meant socialization into subservience; learned helplessness arising from powerlessness; hierarchical structures retaining power in male hands; and patriarchal dominance. Wright (1986) comments that 'nurses are befuddled by confused gender hierarchies (male/doctor dominance, female/nurse subservience) and trapped by the altruism of their calling. If only Florence Nightingale had trained her nurses in assertiveness instead of military obedience to dogma and authority!'

Some feminist writers view nursing as exhibiting some of the characteristics of an oppressed group, including lack of self-esteem, lack of pride in nursing demonstrated in failure to support professional organizations, in addition to displaced aggression towards colleagues, contributing to the persisting inability to achieve consensus on important occupational issues.

Many would vigorously contend against the feminist viewpoint on the problems of nursing in its drive towards professional recognition but the issues raised pose serious questions which can only cause continuing tension if persistently ignored.

In turning from the issues raised by the feminist approach to those relating to the problems of a knowledge base in nursing is again to address a highly contentious subject area. The great majority of sociological studies into professions and professionalism, whether utilizing a trait or functionalist model, cite a body of knowledge as being one of the essential components of a profession.

The slow emergence of a knowledge base in nursing is sometimes ascribed to Florence Nightingale's emphasis on tasks and procedures. Johnson (1974) comments that 'nursing stands today as a field of practice without a scientific heritage – an occupation created by society long ago to offer a distinctive service, but one still ill-defined in practical terms, a profession without the theoretical base it seems to require'.

A professionalizing occupation such as nursing, conscious of its problems in this sphere, seeks development of nursing theory at both basic and complex levels in order better to meet the demands of this dominant criterion. The development of nursing theory, therefore, can be seen as a vehicle of professionalization for nurses.

Nursing theory, it has been suggested, attempts to describe, predict and explain nursing activities, to provide a frame of reference and a foundation for safe practice based on a developing nursing science (Stevens, 1979). The developing and testing of theory should, therefore, remain a high priority in nursing. Some writers also believe that the development of nursing theory may have a positive effect upon the discipline of nursing with respect to the attainment of higher levels of professional education.

There is little doubt that the education of nurses continues to be a highly contentious issue, and this will be more fully addressed in the following chapter. It is therefore sufficient perhaps to note here that certain influences within nursing relating to education have tended to be obstructive to, and restrictive of, the professionalization process in nursing this century. Included here must be the early medical dominance, historically, in training schemes, and the prevailing philosophy of some of the early nurse leaders, encapsulated perhaps in the comment of Catherine Wood in 1880: 'In the training of our nurses we should aim at making them intelligent, conscientious hand-maidens to the medical staff . . .'

A further factor was the obsessive emphasis on obedience. Florence Nightingale viewed professionalization of nurses to some extent in class terms, believing it should enshrine the middle class values for women of that period, such as responsibility, honesty, femininity, and obedience. These qualities, though of value in themselves do not encourage independence or assertiveness.

There also developed, as the years progressed, an anti-academic bias within nursing which is only now beginning to be overcome. One prominent nurse educator has drawn attention to the fact that 'there is widespread suspicion of the "academic" nurse. While the clever doctor or lawyer is spoken of with awe, the clever nurse is usually the subject of sneers and considered unlikely to be any good "practically"' (Chapman, 1974).

Educational entry requirements have remained at a low level and the needs of education, until more recently, have continued to be subservient to the needs of the hospital service. Regrettably some of the strongest resistance to educational change in nursing has come from within the occupation itself. Yet, as has been seen, one of the major hallmarks of a profession is the possession of a systematic body of knowledge. This requires both education and research, neither of which have, as yet, been adequately supported or funded in the British context. Better education would provide increased skills and greater ability to initiate action on the part of nurses. Increased research would assist in building the body of knowledge so essential to the future growth of nursing. A later chapter in this book will examine the field of nursing research in detail.

It would be an omission not to consider the place of the Nursing Process in terms of the professionalization of nursing. A relatively new concept in British nursing, it did not become a subject for debate until the 1970s, having been developed in the United States in the 1960s. Early resistance to it was fairly rapidly overcome in this country and by 1977 implementation was in progress in a number of hospitals.

The Nursing Process, in replacing the task-orientated approach to care, encourages instead a problem-solving, patient-centred approach. It has been suggested that it will bring nursing closer to the professional trait model, enabling the nurse to become an independent practitioner with authority based on nursing knowledge. But for this to occur nursing may need to rid itself of its hand-maiden image and forge new relationships with, and greater independence from the medical profession; moving perhaps to the position of 'colleagueship' advocated by Katz and others. Chapter 3 will examine the problems of integrating theory and practice in the clinical context.

Protagonists of the Nursing Process approach to care see it as instrumental in making the distinction between nursing and medicine clear. Care must utilize a nursing rather than a medical model.

Aspirants to professional status for nurses view the Nursing Process in terms of re-establishing boundaries between qualified and unqualified staff, and of furthering nursing autonomy. It brings about a re-definition of basic care, and the knowledge and skill required for its delivery.

Some writers however have doubts that the Process, designed to enhance standards of care, would necessarily be able also to facilitate increased professional status and autonomy. Already there is evidence of resistance by some members of the medical profession regarding increased autonomy on the part of nurses.

It may be appropriate at this point to consider the problem of autonomy and the future role of the nurse. O'Reilly (1982) makes the point that

'the nursing profession has for too long been viewed as only a support service whose duties were directly dictated by and subordinate to both the physician and the hospital administrator. Rarely defined as a separate entity, an autonomous body with its own skills, areas of expertise, and responsibilities, nursing has suffered the indignities common to many other female-dominated professions – that of role confusion and accompanying diffusion of responsibility'.

McClure (1978) draws attention to the problem of passivity among nurses and comments that nurses seem to be psychologically geared to respond to others rather than initiate action themselves. Reasons for this may well be found to reside in the historical origins of nursing, as well as in terms of the socialization of women. The organizational structure within which the nurse practises may also serve to foster compliance, particularly where negative sanctions are felt to be unduly powerful.

Batey and Lewis (1982), in their study of autonomy, noted that the term had variable uses, including self direction, independence, and not being controlled by an external agent. It cannot be considered either in isolation from responsibility and authority in nursing. However, authority defined as the power to command, or act, or exact obedience may itself be problematic in nursing, involving as it does a multiplicity of factors, including education, expertise, constraints of a bureaucratic framework, and the power and influence of significant other groups.

Batey and Lewis state that once authority is defined as the rightful power to fulfill a responsibility, autonomy becomes the freedom to exercise that rightful power, and that this freedom derives from two sources: the organizational structure and the individual professional, the structure allowing for the exercise of autonomy, and the individual displaying an attitude of willingness to assert and act on decisions seen to be appropriate (Batey and Lewis, 1982). Frequently both these factors can be seen to be missing in current nursing contexts. Subsequent chapters in this book will explore these problems further.

Very little attention has been drawn as yet to the problem of power and politics in modern nursing, and their influence on, and relationship to the process of professionalization. A later chapter will examine this area in some depth and therefore comments here will be limited.

Haralambos (1986) provides a useful, yet simple definition of power: 'power is the ability of an individual or group to realise their aims even if others resist'. In terms of that type of definition it would appear that nursing, as an occupational group, is still wanting in this respect. There is a pressing need for nurses to understand both the nature and the meaning of power, and an awareness that power begets power. Nurses often fail to question who holds or acquires power, and underestimate their own power potential as a group, particularly in terms of weight of numbers, being the largest grouping of health care workers. Disunity within also serves to weaken this potential further. Power is viewed by many writers, both sociologists and nurses, as being an essential element for professionalism. There is currently a continuing need for nurses to become more politically aware. In failing to do so they fail their patients and themselves, while others outside nursing, as so often in the past, make the decisions for them. The need is for greater assertiveness. Unfortunately, as Clay (1987) comments, 'nursing is one of the most unassertive professions in the United Kingdom'.

Changes in society influence the process of professionalization; this is so in nursing as in other occupational groups. Changing social norms and mores, advancing science and technology, the feminist movement, political and economic change, to name but a few, have all exerted an influence on nursing, and the contexts in which it is practised. A health service for all, funded from taxation, has also created new demands and expectations, as well as increased consumer criticism. A subsequent chapter will explore the problems relating to the National Health Service.

Although the role of the nurse continues to be extended and specialized in response to the above factors, over the past two decades the key role of the ward sister/charge nurse has suffered a relative devaluation. In a comparative study, McClosky (1981) commented on the lack of clinical promotion ladders in British nursing, noting that promotion, with its attendant increased remuneration, can only be attained in administration or teaching, effectively removing the individual from the clinical setting at what should be the peak of their professional life. The suggestion has been made that 'the morale of nurses and the standard of nursing are unlikely to be restored until excellence as a ward sister carries corresponding prestige and salary as does excellence as a physician or surgeon' (Royal Society of Medicine and Josiah Macy Jr Foundation, 1973).

Members of the established professions gain personal and

professional reward from direct service to their clients. In nursing both status and increased remuneration are achieved by moving away from the bedside. At a stage when nursing is striving to legitimize its standing as a profession it should be borne in mind that few professions worthy of the name permit their key practitioners to become thus devalued either in terms of status or in terms of material reward.

Many points have been raised relating to the professionalization process in nursing, though within the confines of a single chapter it is not possible to consider every pertinent aspect. Some of the factors considered have perhaps tended to indicate that there exist, and are likely to remain, some formidable barriers to the attainment of true professional status for nurses.

A number of writers and observers of the current nursing scene have sought to enumerate what these problems are. Moloney (1986) cites the following factors as constituting some of the difficulties barring the way:

1. lack of an identifiable knowledge base;
2. problems within the education system;
3. lack of monopoly over nursing services;
4. lack of autonomy.

To this list could be added the problems of internal disunity.

Other commentators, taking a different stance, utter words of warning regarding the long-term wisdom of nursing as an occupation seeking too avidly to approximate to full professional status as it is currently perceived. O'Brien (1978) warns that 'the implicit assumption that professionalism is "good" for society and consequently also for nursing has gone largely unchallenged. In fact professionalism itself does not guarantee improved patient care, and in certain situations the opposite effect may occur'. Salvage (1985), writing in a similar vein, comments that nurses tend to accept uncritically that professionalism means excellence in standards and the protection of the public, while ignoring the negative aspects of greed and élitism. The potential for divisiveness, exclusivity and distancing from other groups of health care workers, thus raising barriers inimical to satisfactory working relationships tend to be overlooked or disregarded.

Nursing is currently at a crucial stage in its development. Powerful arguments for and against the continuance of the professionalization process are frequently put forward, as well as warnings concerning the selection of what are deemed desirable features of professionalism, while encouraging the discarding of what is seen to be inappropriate to nursing. Some would go further and suggest that nurses should stop trying to convince themselves that they are professionals at all.

Some would advocate the approach suggested by Oakley (1984); that nurses should seek to reshape their own place in health care, allying themselves more closely with the self-stated needs of patients, as articulated through the consumer health care movement. She goes on to suggest that much of what is advocated through the movement is already extant in traditional nursing ideology, and that therefore nursing needs only to recover its past.

French (1984) notes that nursing is in the rare position of being able to professionalize while holding the service ethic in a true position of dominance, and poses the question 'why shouldn't nursing become one of the first professions not to abuse this ethic purely for economic gain?'

Nurses may agree or strongly disagree with much of the foregoing, but perhaps would agree that the basic underlying issue is one of seeking greater power and influence; not necessarily for group or individual aggrandisement, but to ensure that the voice of the largest occupational group in health care is heard, and more importantly, listened to. McClosky (1981) comments that a measure of professionalism is only important in that it measures that power. An 'ideal' profession has too much power, a semi-profession has too little.

Nursing needs to consider very carefully indeed the path to power it chooses, and the voices it listens to.

REFERENCES

Ashley, J. (1972) *Hospitals, Paternalism and the Role of the Nurse.* Teachers College Press, New York.

Batey, M.V. and Lewis, F.M. (1982) Clarifying autonomy and accountability in nursing service 1. *Journal of Nursing Administration,* **12**(9) Sep, 13–18.

Becker, H.S. (1962) The nature of a profession, in *Education for the Professions: Sixty First Yearbook of the National Society for the Study of Education, part 2.* University of Chicago Press, Chicago, Ill.

Bevis, E. (1982) *Curriculum Building in Nursing – a Process*, 3rd edn, Mosby, St. Louis, MO.

Carr-Saunders, A.M. and Wilson, P.A. (1933) *The Professions*. Clarendon, Oxford.

Caplow, T.A. (1954) *The Sociology of Work*. University of Minnesota Press, Minneapolis.

Chapman, C. (1974) University education for nurses. *Welsh National School of Medicine*, **1** (1) Jun, 65–6.

Chinn, P.L. and Wheeler, C.E. (1985) Feminism and nursing. *Nursing Outlook*, **33**(2) Mar/Apr 74–7.

Clay, T. (1987) *Nurses, Power and Politics*. Heinemann Nursing, London.

Dingwall, R. and Lewis, P. (eds) (1983) *The Sociology of the Professions*. Macmillan, London.

Elliott, P. (1972) *The Sociology of the Professions*. Macmillan, London.

Etzioni, A. (ed.) (1969) *The Semi-professions and their Organization*. Free Press, New York.

Flexner, A. (1915) Is social work a profession? *School and Society*, **1**, 26 Jun, 901–11.

Freidson, E. (1983) The theory of professions: state of the art, in *The Sociology of the Professions*, (eds) R. Dingwall and P. Lewis Macmillan, London. pp. 19–37.

French, P. (1984) The path to professionalism. *Senior Nurse*, **1**, 2 May, 14–15.

Gamer, M. (1979) The ideology of professionalism. *Nursing Outlook*, **27**(2) Feb, 108–11.

Goode, W. (1969) The theoretical limits of professionalism. In *The Semi-professions and Their Organization* (ed. A. Etzioni), Free Press, New York.

Habenstein, R.W. and Christ, E.A. (1955) *Professionalizer, Traditionalizer and Utilizer*. University of Missouri Press, Columbia, MO.

Hall, C. (1980) The nature of nursing and the education of the nurse. *Journal of Advanced Nursing*, **5**(2), 149–59.

Haralambos, M. (1986) *Sociology – a New Approach*, 2nd edn, Causeway, Ormskirk.

Heraud, B. (1973) Professionalism, radicalism and social change, in *Professionalisation and Social Change* (ed. P. Halmos), University of Keele, Keele. (University of Keele monograph 20)

Illich, I. (1977) *Disabling Professions*. Marion Boyars, London.

Johnson, D.E. (1974) Development of theory: a requisite for nursing as a primary health profession. *Nursing Research*, **23**(5) Sep/Oct, 372–7.

Johnson, M. (1978) Auxiliaries: nursing auxiliaries and nurse professionalization. *Nursing Times*, **74**, 23 Feb, 313–17.

Johnson, T. (1972) *Professions and Power*. Macmillan, London.

Katz, F.E. (1969) Nurses, in *The Semi-professions and Their Organization* (ed. A. Etzioni), Free Press, New York.

Larson, M.S. (1977) *The Rise of Professionalism*. University of California Press, Berkeley, CA.

McClosky, J.C. (1981) The professionalization of nursing: United States and England. *International Nursing Review*, **28**(2) Mar/Apr, 40–7.

McClure, M.L. (1978) The long road to accountability. *Nursing Outlook*, **26**(1) Jan, 47–50.

Maresh, J. (1986) *Women's History, Nursing History: Parallel Stories.* Yale University Press, New Haven, CT.

Melosh, B. (1982) *The Physicians Hand: Nurses and Nursing in the Twentieth Century.* Temple University Press, Philadelphia, PA.

Millerson, G. (1964a) Dilemmas of professionalism. *New Society*, **3**, 4 Jun, 15–18.

Millerson, G. (1964b) *The Qualifying Associations.* Routledge and Kegan Paul, London.

Moloney, M. (1986) *Professionalization of Nursing.* Lippincott, Philadelphia.

Nightingale, F. (1860) *Notes on Nursing: What it is and What it is not.* Harrison, London.

Oakley, A. (1984) What price professionalism? The importance of being a nurse. *Nursing Times*, **80**, 12 Dec, 24–7.

O'Brien, D. (1978) Professionalism in perspective. *Nursing Times*, **74**, 15 Jun, 990.

O'Reilly, D.P. (1982) Toward autonomy of the nursing profession. *Nursing Leadership*, **5**(3) Sep, 18–22.

Parsons, M. (1986) The profession in a class by itself. *Nursing Outlook*, **34**(6) Nov/Dec. 270-5.

Pinch, W.J. (1981) Feminine attributes in a masculine world. *Nursing Outlook*, **29**(10) Oct, 596–9.

Royal Society of Medicine and Josiah Macy Jr Foundation (1973) *The Greater Medical Profession.* The Foundation, New York.

Salvage, J. (1985) *The Politics of Nursing.* Heinemann Nursing, London.

Speedy, S. (1987) Feminism and the professionalization of nursing. *Australian Journal of Advanced Nursing*, **4**(2) Dec/Feb, 20–8.

Stevens, B. (1979) *Nursing Theory, Analysis, Application, Evaluation.* Little, Brown, Boston.

Vollmer, H.W. and Mills, D.J. (eds.) (1966) *Professionalization.* Prentice-Hall, Englewood Cliffs, NJ.

White, R. (1982) Back to basics. *Nursing Times*, **78**, 27 Oct, 1796–7.

White, R. (1984) Altruism is not enough: barriers in the development of nursing as a profession. *Journal of Advanced Nursing*, **9**(6) Nov, 555–62.

Wilensky, H.L. (1964) The professionalization of everyone? *American Journal of Sociology*, **70**(2) Sep, 137–58.

Wood, C. (1880) *A Handbook of Nursing for the Home and the Hospital.* Cassell, London.

Wright, S. (1986) Power, professions and practice. *Nursing Practice*, **1**(3), 135–7.

BIBLIOGRAPHY

Davies, C. (1976) Experience of dependency and control in work: the case of nurses. *Journal of Advanced Nursing*, **1**(4) Jul, 273–82.

Davies, C. (1977) Continuities in the development of hospital nursing in Britain. *Journal of Advanced Nursing*, **2**(5) Sep, 479–93.

De Santis, G. (1982) Power, tactics and the professionalization process. *Nursing and Health Care*, **3**(1) Jan 14–17, 24.

Fawcett, J. (1984) The metaparadigm of nursing: present status and future refinements. *Image*, **16**(3) Summer, 84–9.

Hector, W. (1973) *The Work of Mrs Bedford Fenwick and the Rise of Professional Nursing*. Royal College of Nursing, London.

2 Nursing education – a luxury or necessity?

PETA ALLAN

To be educated is not to have arrived,
it is to travel with a different view
Peters (1965)

Nursing education is poised on the brink of unprecedented change. Such change is essential and results from a lack of action despite many attempts at reform. To many, nursing education is a luxury and as such, is treated with low priority status. This is particularly evident at present when health services strive to increase scarce resources to meet essential elements of direct care provision.

Most of those involved with health care would admit that some nursing education is essential, but only a few have given careful consideration to the detail of the present position of preparation for nursing. The latter group acknowledges that a number of reports have been produced which demonstrate that nurses are ill prepared to undertake the practice and responsibilities of nursing. The recent reports have raised the profession's awareness of the many interrelated issues surrounding nursing education and revitalized the discussion on them. Although many of these issues had previously been well documented, these previous reports produced little action. However, many people now recognize that the present preparation of nurses is not cost effective for employers, employees, managers or consumers of the health service. So how should these fundamental issues be addressed?

Certainly, the debate on nursing education in the United Kingdom has never before been so loud or so clear, and the profession is demanding change. A number of new Reports have intensified and informed the debate. In 1984, the United Kingdom Central Council for Nursing, Midwifery and Health Visiting (UKCC) set up a study 'To determine the education and training required in preparation for the professional practice of nursing, midwifery and health visiting in relation to the projected health care needs in the 1990s and beyond and to make recommendations.' This work which became known as Project 2000, was remitted to the UKCC Educational Policy Advisory Committee (EPAC) under the Chairmanship of Miss Margaret Green. In the process of undertaking the study, six Project Papers were produced and widely discussed by EPAC members and UKCC officers with the nursing, midwifery and health visiting professions. Further work was undertaken by EPAC and in 1986, the Project 2000 Report *A New Preparation for Practice* was presented to the UKCC. It was agreed that the Report be issued for wide consultation.

During the consultation period, detailed work was undertaken on specific aspects of the Report's recommendations including the costs and benefits. The professions responded to the consultation in great number and with a high level of agreement to the recommendations. On receipt of the detailed work and the professions' response, the UKCC considered and agreed final proposals which were presented, with the Chairmen of the four National Boards, to Health Departments' Ministers in February 1987. Ministerial consultation began in March and was finally completed in September 1987.

In May 1988, the Secretary of State for Social Services, John Moore, wrote to the Chairman of the UKCC giving the Government's response to the proposals. The need for change was endorsed by the Government, together with agreement, in principle, to the changes proposed.

The Royal College of Nursing (RCN) and the English National Board for Nursing, Midwifery and Health Visiting (ENB) have each made a major contribution to the debate on nursing education. The report of the RCN Commission on Nursing Education *The Education of Nurses : A New Dispensation*, and the ENB Consultation Paper, *Professional Education/Training Courses*, were published in 1985. These documents were widely discussed and a growing awareness of the need for change in the current provision of nursing education emerged.

Pre-registration nursing programmes should enable students to learn how to nurse, but it is questionable whether such existing programmes achieve this purpose. In the past, this preparation has been almost entirely hospital based with an emphasis on ill health, tasks and procedures. The importance of including the use of nursing models, clinical research, primary nursing and health promotion in nursing programmes has been advocated (Pembrey, 1985). Where these are included, they enable the nurse to provide advice, support and care for individual patients or clients and family/friends, dependent on their physical, mental and social needs. Therefore, all nursing preparation should be devised to permit additional learning both for advances in particular areas of practice and in order to meet rapidly changing health needs. Many nurses require specific post-registration education to undertake particular roles. A range of programmes exists and subjects include clinical specialties, health promotion, management and teaching. However, such post-registration education is often seen as a luxury.

Several of the problems in the provision of effective nursing education result from the inter-dependence of education with the provision of a nursing service. Patient services have relied heavily on student nurses being part of the labour force. All too often it is students and unqualified staff who provide nursing care in hospitals rather than this being directed/given by qualified nurses. The far-reaching effects of the inappropriate use of staff are now being acknowledged as registered nurses leave because of lack of job satisfaction and students fail to complete their education programmes because of stress resulting from a lack of appropriate preparation; it is a vicious circle (Figure 2.1). In many parts of the United Kingdom, this vicious circle exacerbates the high intake and high wastage of nursing staff. Figure 2.2 shows the size of the problem on a UK basis.

It is essential to build and maintain a pool of qualified and experienced nurses and teachers who are able to provide care, assist students to learn, and act as role models. Without such a pool, little progress can be made in the provision of appropriate nursing education to prepare nurses to provide improved patient and client care.

Despite the problems which exist, there have been some important developments in the provision of nursing education over

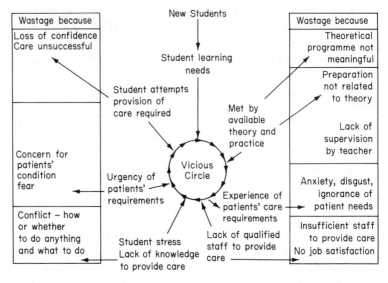

Figure 2.1 Factors creating the present vicious circle.

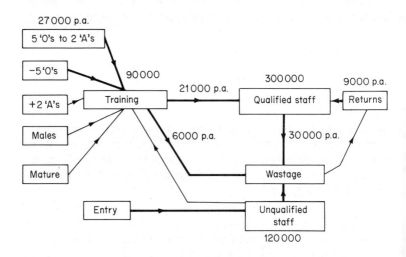

Source: From the UKCC Report on the costs, benefits and manpower implications of Project 2000 undertaken by Price Waterhouse.

Figure 2.2 The National Health Service nursing workforce simplified manpower model.

the past 25 years. To some extent, these have been the result of changes in the requirements of statutory bodies, international influences, the growth of nurse teachers' knowledge of education, the determination and enthusiasm of individuals at the local level, or a combination of all or some of these. Such developments include: the introduction of assessments in practical settings; the broadening of practical experience requirements; programmes of concurrent theory and practice which provide meaningful 'add on' learning; experimental programmes, for example programmes which lead to more than one professional qualification, and programmes where the examinations are completed by the end of the second year of a three-year preparation; the establishment of colleges of nursing/midwifery; partnerships between schools or colleges of nursing and colleges of higher education; an increase in shared learning between nurses, midwives and health visitors and with students of other disciplines; the use of specialist teachers from subjects allied to nursing; the growth in knowledge of curriculum renewal activites; the importance of a dynamic curriculum which incorporates health promotion, health trends and issues in a qualitative and relevant way, rather than disease and cure dominated, and, the growth of open learning.

In some parts of the United Kingdom, these initiatives have been more successful than others. The fluctuation in the numbers of suitable applicants to nursing education has influenced the types and levels of the programmes offered. In this context it is interesting to note the present low number of programmes for part-time students and the lack of provision of programmes for mature students, despite the success of the Portsmouth Scheme (Hooper, 1985). The supply and demand issue is clearly seen in relation to the preparation of nurses for entry to second level parts of the register. When there is a good supply of applicants to first level nurse programmes the numbers accepted for second level nurse preparations fall, and vice versa.

SELECTION OF STUDENTS

Many issues on the selection of students for entry to nursing programmes remain unresolved. Valid and reliable tools are required to measure an applicant's ability to complete the nursing education programme successfully, to indicate the potential for success in the practice of nursing and to demonstrate a commitment to a career in nursing. At present there is no evidence to suggest that such tools exist. The current statutory requirements for entry to first level nursing programmes are concerned with a candidate's age and educational qualifications. The age of entry '. . . shall be not less than seventeen and one half years of age on the first day of the commencement of a course except that in exceptional circumstances related to specific courses the Council on the recommendation of a Board may agree to entry earlier but in no circumstances at less than seventeen years of age' (Statutory Instrument 1983 No. 873, The Nurse Midwives and Health Visitors Rules Approval Order, Nurse Training Rule 15).

Since 1 January 1986, the minimum educational requirements for entry to first level nurse programmes throughout the United Kingdom has been five subjects at pass standard in a UK certificate of education at ordinary level, or overseas equivalent, or a specified pass standard in one of the three DC Tests approved by the UKCC (Statutory Instrument 1983 No. 873 Rule 16(1)). In 1987, a second level nurse qualification, in specified circumstances, was added to the entry routes in the Statutory Instrument 1987 No. 446 The Nurses, Midwives and Health Visitors (Entry to Training Requirements) Amendment Rules Approval Order, Nurse Training Rule 16(3). In 1988, the UKCC agreed to widen the entry gate by including national vocational qualifications and educational criteria approved by the UKCC as an additional route.

Dodd (1973) demonstrated a positive correlation between the number of passes in the General Certificate of Education (England and Wales) and success in the final examination for entry to first level parts of the register. This is hardly surprising given that until recently, the types of examinations for both qualifications were similar. It is difficult to find evidence to justify the present traditional educational requirements in terms of their relevance to success in the practice of nursing.

Those who select students have, in the past, relied heavily on their personally favoured criteria for selection. The interview, with all its well-documented deficiencies, has been widely used. Specific subject passes in school leaving examinations have often been required, and the number of pass grades has ranged from the minimum required by the UKCC to that required for university entrance.

The historical perspective of educational entry requirements has been described by White (1985) as a means of recruiting nurses and de-skilling nursing. The supply and demand issue again raises its head! At present, a number of research projects are being undertaken on specific aspects of the selection process; these raise many questions. Are educational qualifications indicators of success, or a means of attempting to secure academic currency for nursing qualifications? Are there valid and reliable measures which are indicators of motivation and commitment to nursing? Should these other tools be used alone or in combination with educational achievements? Is success in a specific test the most appropriate route of entry for all entrants to nursing? Can factors in those registered nurses who are successfully practising be identified, and are these factors measurable in persons prior to their undertaking a nursing programme? These are some of the issues currently being addressed by researchers. It will be interesting to see the results of this work as well as the outcomes resulting from the recent widening of the entry gate.

Selecting persons for nursing is one thing, retaining them in the profession is another. It may be argued that if the former were more appropriate than at present, the high intake and high wastage scenario in Figure 2.2 would not occur. But it is occurring and, as indicated earlier, clearly has a negative effect on the provision of nursing education.

THE GAP BETWEEN THEORY AND PRACTICE

One of the main causes of frustration and dissatisfaction leading to wastage of students and registered nurses is the gap between the theory taught in the classroom, and the actual practice in clinical settings. This problem exists in many parts of Europe as well as in the United Kingdom. The need to seek creative and sound ways of reducing this gap, was identified by a Working Part of the European Community Advisory Committee on Training in Nursing. The group has identified reasons for the existence of the gap, and work is continuing on ways in which it could be reduced.

The reasons in part arise from historical factors. In many cases there has been a separation between those providing the teaching of nurses and those undertaking nursing. This has led to emphasis on a theoretical approach by teachers, often from out-dated knowledge of the practice of nursing. Additionally, teachers have been required to teach aspects of practice in which they have never had clinical experience. In some instances, this has created insecurity in teachers and reluctance to undertake teaching in clinical settings. Likewise, many clinical nurses feel unprepared for a teaching role and are, therefore, reluctant to combine this with their direct patient care.

Nursing knowledge, and subjects allied to nursing, are expanding at an increasing rate. It is difficult for teachers to remain up to date over the wide range of subjects in the nursing curriculum. And yet, teaching based on up-to-date knowledge and research is essential for effective learning.

Until recently, the emphasis has been on task-oriented nursing. In the past few years, there have been positive attempts to consider the process of nursing in the context of the total care of the individual. The latter gives meaning to that which students are learning; continued existence of the former enlarges the gap between theory and practice.

Reference to the reliance on student labour has already been made; in many situations, students are used in practical settings as 'pairs of hands'. This emphasis on students' presence for their service commitment, as opposed to their educational needs, often results in gaps in experience and the absence of an appropriate link between theory and practice.

Narrowing the gap between theory and practice would assist in the reduction of student wastage, the loss of qualified staff and thus, improve nursing education and patient and client care.

STUDENT STATUS

Perhaps the most contentious issue in pre- and post-registration education is the status of students. The vast majority of nursing programmes in the United Kindom involve a substantial service contribution, which is currently estimated on a United King-

dom basis as 60% of the three-year programme. Whilst it ι
acknowledged that nursing cannot be learned in isolation from the
reality of care provision, it must be emphasized that exposure to,
and working in, practical settings, does not of itself equate with learning how to nurse and how to accept responsibility for practice.

The majority of entrants to nursing preparation are 18-year-old
girls whose previous experience of life may have been confined to
that gained in association with their family and friends; in many
instances this experience is not extensive. In the present system,
students undergo a four to eight week preparation as an introduction to working in the National Health Service, and as a brief
preparation for their role. Students are then placed in ward settings
where they function as full-time employees. There may be adequate supervision and guidance available some of the time but, in a
growing number of instances, not all of the time. Is this so-called
apprenticeship training (so called because an apprenticeship
usually implies one learner to one qualified person, and this does
not pertain) an appropriate way of providing care to people who
require competent nursing care? Equally, is this treatment of
students likely to motivate and inform their nursing? There can be
no other occupational group where such responsibility is placed on
unprepared staff. Patients are often unaware of the students'
inexperience or lack of knowledge, and seek assistance far beyond
the students' capabilities. Why does the student not recognize his
or her inadequacies to provide support or care needed and refuse
to attempt to meet patients' needs? If he or she is the only person
present, is it possible to walk away and disregard such need?
Indeed, the very processes at work will socialize the student into
accepting that when care is required it must be given. A number of
writers have raised serious questions about the present practices,
Ogier (1981), Fretwell (1982) and Gott (1984), question how the
student can learn and be a full member of the ward team.

Conversely, it would be totally inappropriate to provide nursing
education which did not prepare a nurse to undertake care and to
accept responsibility for such care. The crucial point here is that
care giving and responsibility should only be accepted by the nurse
following appropriate preparation.

The Project 2000 proposals included supernumerary status for
students during the three-year preparation as an essential element
in effective preparation for practice. During the proposed

arning would take place in a variety of practical
student occupying an observer, participant obser-
t role as was appropriate to the stage of learning.
the fact that some of the care given would be of
ue to service, as opposed to adding to the quality of care
provided, a service contribution of 20% was identified. However,
the total programme should be educationally led and be provided
in such a way as to prevent the student experiencing reality shock
on its successful completion. Appropriate preparation and a
carefully controlled transition from student to competent nurse is
essential to provide effective practice.

The scale of the manpower and cost implications of such a
change are considerable. A range of supportive management
action, and increased government resources are required to establish qualified providers of care, before student labour can be
withdrawn. Thus, the implementation of such a scheme will need
to be phased so that standards of care provided for patients and
clients are not lowered. There is a need for fundamental change in
the attitudes of many employers including those related to part-
time work and provision of child-care facilities; there are hard
political decisions on allocation of resources to be made. But while
many are wondering 'how' such changes can be achieved, most
who have become informed on the complexity and seriousness of
the present situation accept the need to change the present status
of the student.

NURSING COMPETENCE

Meaningful selection and supernumerary status of students are
essential for the effective preparation of safe, confident nurses who
are able to provide a high standard of care, in a range of settings,
and be accountable for that care.

In the past, assumptions have been made that by placing
emphasis on the content of nursing education programmes, competence to nurse and high standards of care would be achieved.
Early documentation from the statutory bodies responsible for
the training of nurses included detailed lists of hours for
particular subjects, and specific placements which must be included

in the training programmes.

In England and Wales the 1969 syllabus for General Nurses introduced a major move away from this approach. Prescription gave way to principles to be addressed, and details of practice required were replaced by broad experience categories. But the emphasis remained on process; a belief was held that exposure to the required 'treatment' led to success in examinations, which in turn led to 'good' nurses who were accountable for their practice. The parameters of practice, and the professional competence achieved by the preparation, remained undefined.

In the early 1970s, Bendall (1975) drew attention to the absence of linkage between the successful completion of nurse training and the successful practice of nursing. Work began on identifying nursing competence. In 1974 The General Nursing Council for England and Wales produced *A Specification of Nursing Competence*. This paper was intended to provide a broad specification of nursing to cover both the mental illness and general care fields, and serve as a basis for considering the objectives of training. The major sections were on observation, interpretation, planning, action and evaluation.

This prompted varying degrees of activity among nurse teachers on the development of behavioural objectives which previously had been little used in nursing education. The need to specify the activity to be learned, and the standard of performance, became widely acknowledged. Much detailed work was done, but difficulties emerged in the formulation of behavioural objectives in the affective domain and on the principles of nursing practice. Such difficulties led, in some cases, to the abandonment of this route of identification, quantification and measurement of learning, in favour of a return to the process approach. However, the excursion into these 'territories' was sufficient to demonstrate to many the wisdom of this approach. The need to identify clearly the behaviour necessary for professional practice as a registered nurse became established. It was in this climate, that the new UKCC Nurse Training Rules were drafted in 1983; these define the competencies required prior to registration as a nurse based on the framework of content carried over from the former statutory bodies.

Rule 18(1) of the Statutory Instrument 1983, No. 873, requires first level nurses to have undertaken courses which

. . . shall enable an application to be made for admission to Part 1, 3, 5 or 8 of the register and shall provide opportunities to enable the student to accept responsibility for her personal professional development and to acquire the competencies to: advise on the promotion of health and the prevention of illness; recognise situations that may be detrimental to the health and well being of the individual; carry out those activities involved when conducting the comprehensive assessment of a person's nursing requirements; recognise the significance of the observations made and use these to develop an initial nursing assessment; devise a plan of nursing care based on the assessment with the co-operation of the patient, to the extent that this is possible, taking into account the medical prescription; implement the planned programme of nursing care and where appropriate teach and co-ordinate other members of the caring team who may be responsible for implementing specific aspects of the nursing care; review the effectiveness of the nursing care provided, and where appropriate, initiate any action that may be required; work in a team with other nurses, and with medical and para-medical staff and social workers; undertake the management of the care of a group of patients over a period of time and organise the appropriate support services; related to the care of the particular type of patient with whom she is likely to come in contact when registered in that Part of the register for which the student intends to qualify.

A clear distinction was made between the competencies required for practice as a first level nurse, compared with practice as a second level (enrolled) nurse.

The same Statutory Instrument requires that courses for second level nurses shall

. . . be designed to prepare the student to undertake nursing care under the direction of a person registered in Part 1, 3, 5 or 8 of the register and provide opportunities for the student to develop the competencies required to: assist in carrying out comprehensive observation of the patient and help in assessing her care requirements; develop skills to enable her to assist in the implementation of nursing care under the direction of a person registered in Part 1, 3, 5 or 8 of the register; accept delegated nursing tasks; assist in reviewing the effectivness of the care provided; work in a team with other nurses and with medical and para-medical staff and social workers; related to the care of the particular type of patient with whom she is likely to come into contact when registered in that Part of the register for which the student intends to qualify.

The change in approach indicated by the style of Rule 18 received a mixed response from the professions. The pro-process people considered it insufficient to ensure United Kingdom standards. The behavioural objective protagonists considered it contained insufficient detail for parity of national registration levels, favouring a clearer enunciation of definitive behaviours which characterized competence. To some it enabled innovation in the provision of programmes leading to registration whilst ensuring a UK minimum requirement of the kind, standard and content of courses by virtue of the continuation of pre-July 1983 requirements.

This change in emphasis from process to competency encouraged nurses to obtain a clearer understanding of the concept of competence. Performance can be conceptualized as the ability to undertake care to agreed and approved standards. Competency can be defined as the ability to apply knowledge and skills with understanding and the appropriate attitude to specific activities and responsibilities.

Concept of Competency

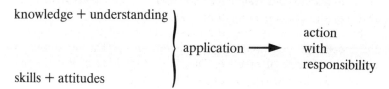

knowledge + understanding

skills + attitudes

application ⟶ action with responsibility

Work has continued on clarifying aspects of competencies required for registration as a nurse. In the UKCC Project 2000 Report *A New Preparation for Practice* (1986) the functioning of the proposed new registered practitioner was described using competencies. These have been refined; and further work has been undertaken to clarify the standards of professional competence required for registration with the UKCC set in the context of the kind, standard and content of the new programmes.

It is essential that all registration programmes meet a UK minimum. The proposed approach would enable innovative nursing programmes to be developed at the local level whilst ensuring that students achieve clearly stated standards of professional competence. A clear description of registration standards is also of value in informing the professions and the public on expectations of the practice and accountability of registered nurses.

An important aspect of designing programmes to achieve the requirements for registration is that this is done by a group of nurse teachers, practitioners and nurse managers. There is often confusion in these groups as to which aspects of the programme have priority and there is a need to achieve a consensus on what is relevant to the education for the practice and responsibility of nursing.

A clear statement of the standards of competence to be achieved for registration is essential if these are to be meaningful for the individual student to measure his or her progress and to serve as a basis for formal evaluation of performance standards.

EDUCATION BEYOND REGISTRATION

In the United Kingdom

Registration follows the successful completion of a nursing programme. Many nurses have viewed registration as the end of their education and training rather than the end of one stage of learning and the beginning of another.

Since the early seventies there has been a growing awareness of the need for additional post-registration clinical learning for particular aspects of practice. The knowledge base of nursing has expanded and new specialties have been developed which require additional learning beyond pre-registration programmes. Such learning has received some attention but the provision of post-registration learning for certain aspects of practice has been minimal. In a number of cases this has resulted in a nursing work force undertaking care from an out of date knowledge base and without the benefit of recent nursing research findings, to aid practice.

There are many nurses who return to work following a break in practice of several years and do not undertake any professional up-dating. Practices may have changed considerably during their non-practising period but the myth that nursing competence, once achieved, remains forever pertinent strongly exists. Are such people competent to nurse? Why is little thought or emphasis given to maintaining valuable nursing competence?

This situation is slowly changing; there is some evidence of an attitude change occurring in employers and employees. At present there is a shortage of qualified nursing staff, and some provision is being made for those returning after a break to be prepared for their return to practice. There is no statutory requirement for this provision for nurses, but an increasing number of employing authorities are realizing the wisdom of providing such learning opportunities. In some instances nurses are requesting re-entry programmes, are prepared to wait for a place on a programme before recommencing work, and are willing to meet the costs of the programme personally. This acceptance of accountability for standards of practice is a major step forward.

Nevertheless, in a survey undertaken by the UKCC in April 1988, it was found that only 8% of NHS employing authorities who responded required a nurse to undertake preparation for return to practice. In the light of the findings of the survey, the UKCC re-affirmed its policy of moving towards a statutory requirement for re-entry programmes for nurses who have a career break and return to practice.

When the nursing, midwifery and health visiting professions were consulted on periodic payment of registration fees, many expressed the view that such payment should be linked with the provision by those practising of evidence of undertaking activities to maintain or improve their practice. The implementation of a requirement to enforce this is complex. Many questions were raised in the UKCC Discussion Document *Mandatory Periodic Refreshment for Nurses and Health Visitors* which was widely circulated to the professions in August 1987.

The Discussion Document suggested that the outcomes of refreshment activities might be:

stimulation of the individual to assess his or her educational needs and take responsibility for his or her own continuing education; promotion of professional growth and development; advancement of theoretical and practical knowledge in the area(s) of practice and in the biological, psychological and sociological aspects of caring; extension of the understanding of research, and its application to the individual's practice; an increase in knowledge of recent legislation which may affect his or her practice.

The response to the discussion with the professions showed agreement to the need for periodic refreshment but a lack of consensus on whether such education activities should be mandatory or voluntary. Advantages and disadvantages of each type of provision were stated. It has been argued that as professional nurses the responsibility for these activities comes within this professional remit and, therefore, no mandate is necessary. Others consider that without a mandate the provision of appropriate activities for such a large occupational group would not be achieved.

In North America

A debate similar to that on periodic refreshment in the United Kingdom has continued in the United States of America for many years. Individual states have adopted different approaches and consideration of these has informed the discussion in the United Kingdom. The present overall provision can be described using five models.

The Commercial Model

The majority of hospitals in the USA operate as commercial organizations. In view of this, considerable emphasis is placed on the need for cost-effective practitioners. The provision of continuing education is perceived as having a dual purpose; the primary one to produce a more competent practitioner, thus improving the efficiency of the hospital on a cost basis; the secondary one, the prestige associated with the provision of a comprehensive range of continuing education programmes. In this model, programmes may be associated with specific aspects of nursing activity within specialty areas of nursing. The value of the programme may be limited to the particular place of employment, as there may be no local or State discussion of content or its regulation. Each learning package is devised to meet the specific activities required by a particular employer.

The Negotiated Model

Some states, and parts of other states are more heavily unionized than others. Many places of employment in unionized areas operate 'association protection', that is the inclusion of a minimum number of hours for continuing education in a nurse's contract of employment. This time period is negotiated at the local level by special departments of the State Nurses' Association/Health and Government Employers Associations or other trade unions.

The activities undertaken in the agreed time periods vary considerably, and are usually determined by the individual based on the availability of continuing education programmes.

The Voluntary Model

The American Nurses' Association has no official view on whether continuing education should be mandatory or voluntary. It is interesting to note that the American Medical Association is against mandatory continuing education. In some of the states which have mandatory continuing education there has been debate on whether this should be rescinded, the main reasons being the difficulty of administering and evaluating the system effectively.

Conversely, many nurses in states which have voluntary continuing education are working to achieve mandatory continuing education. The main reason given for this is the perceived rise in the status of continuing education which would result. However, there are also strong protagonists for voluntary continuing education. The Illinois Nurses' Association in a Resolution on Voluntary Continuing Education in 1983, refers to the fact that, 'The nursing profession has traditionally upheld the concept of individual accountability and responsibility for maintaining competency in practice' and 'Urge nurses to take responsibility for their own training and ... acknowledge that the voluntary approach is a viable means to continued professional learning'.

Similarly, the American Hospital Association firmly supports the policy of voluntary continuing education. After consideration of the findings of the Special Committee on Continued Competence of Health Care Professionals, the Association published a Landmark Statement (1979), which stated its view that it is the responsibility of the individual professional to maintain his or her competence. In summary, the Association stated,

It is obvious that establishing a mandatory continuing education program for licence renewal is not simple. Much time, effort and money will be required to produce a workable system, which, in the long run, still may not be able to protect the public against incompetent practitioners. It is difficult, if not impossible, to legislate learning and its subsequent application. For this reason, and because little evidence currently exists that continuing education in and of itself ensures continued competence, the American Hospital Association, in the interest of quality patient care at a reasonable cost, continues to support and promote voluntary continuing education of health care professionals.

The Mandatory Model

As stated earlier, sixteen states currently require continuing education for re-licensure. Each of these State Boards of Registered Nursing, issue laws relating to Nursing Education licensure – Practice with Rules and Regulations. In California, for example, detailed matters related to continuing education appear in legislation. These include:

- definitions of 'Continuing Education, 'Course', 'Content Relevant to the Practice of Nursing', 'Independent/Home Study Courses', 'Hour' and 'Approved Providers';
- License Renewal Requirements which contain details of time scales, renewal fees, form of proof of satisfactory completion of the stated thirty hours of continuing education;
- expiration of licences – procedures;
- Continuing Education Courses – giving information on those activities deemed to meet the requirements;
- exemption from continuing education requirements stating certain circumstances where the thirty hours are not required;
- Approved Providers giving details of who may offer courses which are considered appropriate for re-licensure;
- continuing education hours – how the thirty hours may be obtained;
- Instructor Qualifications;
- Course Verification;
- advertisement and withdrawal of approval.

The legislation requires that the content of all courses must be relevant to the practice of nursing and specifically must:

(a) be related to the scientific knowledge *and/or* technical skills required for the practice of nursing, or
(b) be related to direct *and/or* indirect *patient/client* care.
(c) Learning experiences are up-dated to enhance the knowledge of the Registered Nurse at a level above that required for licensure.

The State Board of Nursing controls the quality of providers by issuing provider numbers which are obtained by submitting evidence of educationally sound offerings. In 1978, there were 300 bona fide providers in California; by 1984, this number had risen to 4000.

The lists and contents of courses being provided shows a varied range of provision. It is not clear how the content of some of the courses is relevant to the practice of nursing. The difficulties of providing effective control of quality at State Board of Nursing level are clear. A large team of appropriately qualified personnel would be required to undertake this work effectively.

The Military Model

It is the policy of the United States army to recruit registered nurses who have undertaken a baccalaureate degree in nursing. Therefore, as well as being a distinct group of nurses they are also from similar educational backgrounds. It is perhaps this background which has developed the life-long learning approach which exists in the systems of continuing education in use, and in staff members' individual commitment to continuing education.

The army nurses are registered with different State Boards, some require continuing education for re-licensure, others do not. This in no way affects the provision or demand from army nurses for continuing education.

There are several facets to the establishment and progress of this model. Prior to its implementation a study was undertaken to identify the professional and educational requirements for particular posts; a review of these requirements is undertaken on a two-yearly basis. Persons are appointed to particular posts based on experience and formal learning. On employment, any gaps in the individual's ability compared with the requirements of the post are identified. An appropriate compensating programme is undertaken which includes theory and practice. This is followed by a six month part-time course in the area of practice in which the nurse is working.

For appointment to the position of head nurse, a higher degree is required. Nurses are seconded to undertake appropriate higher degrees to add to their clinical experience and knowledge.

The salaries of army nurses are higher than those of nurses employed in civilian hospitals; this has been suggested as one of the reasons why recruitment to army nursing is good. Nurses are employed on a three year contract. During this time, an evaluation of their work performance is made, and opportunity is given to resolve any unmet professional needs with appropriate continuing education. The renewal of a contract is based on the standard of the nurse's performance.

The army anticipate that nurses will require to undertake at least twenty hours of planned continuing education per year. The actual processes undertaken may be proposed by the nurse, or result from advice from his or her senior officer. In making the initial request, the nurse completes a form which includes details of the proposed educational activity and how this will assist his or her performance. The request is processed through the management structure for comment on suitability, but there is no power to veto at middle management level. The form is considered by the Head of the Continuing Education Division and a recommendation made to the Colonel in Chief for Nursing.

The activity requested may be additional experience, an educational programme in the same or another hospital, a formal programme in the state, or in another state. On completion of the activity, the nurse makes a formal presentation to her peers on the knowledge gained.

The partnership between service and education staff in the provision of continuing education is very evident in this model and is a major factor in its success.

Clearly some aspects of these five models overlap, but each is unique in its main approach to continuing education and the maintenance of competence. Several of the models have facets which should be explored in the United Kingdom context.

The United Kingdom Direction

In the professions' response to the UKCC consultation on periodic relicensing (1983), *Funding the Work of the UKCC* and to the Project 2000 Report, periodic continuing education for nursing was clearly seen as a necessity to provide effective standards of care. The present provision is varied, and the steps to improve this situation are complex. The professions have been engaged in wide debate on this subject, in response to the UKCC Discussion Document *Mandatory Periodic Refreshment for Nurses and Health Visitors* but it is clear that there are many issues yet to be resolved. A large number of discussions have been held throughout the United Kingdom and the professions have demonstrated their recognition of the importance of this matter by their overwhelming number of responses to the Discussion Document. After consideration of these responses, the UKCC decided in May 1988 that further work was required before firm decisions could be taken on the appropriate way forward.

THE NEED FOR A DIFFERENT VIEW

The purpose of nursing education is to develop an individual's knowledge skills and attitudes to meet the needs of patients and clients. It is also about leadership, both on a personal level, and to encourage and enable others to develop their abilities to meet the public's needs and the needs of the profession. Therefore, if appropriate standards of care are to be provided, programmes for registration must be meaningful and prepare competent nurses, and this valuable nursing resource must be maintained by additional learning. As indicated in the previous section, continuing education in the United Kingdom has been a rather hit and miss affair, with provision and opportunities varying widely; this situation must be corrected.

Many issues in nursing education remain unresolved. This chapter has included but a few of the many. But the same question is pertinent to all of them. How will the profession itself respond to the challenge which they represent? The Government has endorsed the proposals for educational reform as set out in Project 2000. These include: the need for pre-registration preparation to enable the nurse to practise in institutional and non-institutional settings; the provision of an eighteen-month common foundation programme for all student nurses followed by a further eighteen-month programme in nursing of the adult, the child, persons with mental handicap or in mental health; the need for students to have supernumerary status for the greater part of their time and receive non-means tested NHS bursaries; the move towards one new level of registered nurse; the development of a range of support workers; and the widening of the entry gate to nursing programmes. However, no progress will be made unless the nursing, midwifery and health visiting professions take action to further the work needed to make these proposals a reality.

At the local level improvements can be made in many places and within existing resources to start the process of change. Adequate preparation of those already qualified is essential for success. Attitudes to learning, and sharing of learning experiences, can be developed and built upon. A questioning approach to the status quo is essential for the development of initiatives for more effective provision of education. In the past, it has been too easy to wait for Briggs or Project 2000, but the initiative is now clearly with the profession for policy change at the United Kingdom level. Debate should be undertaken to clarify issues with the policy makers at both local and national levels. Progress can be achieved by the provision of a logical and clear presentation of the options. But to achieve this, the internal struggles in the profession, which have waged for so long, must be set aside.

Nursing education is poised on the brink of change, but will the change become reality? Unity of purpose is an essential prerequisite. With such unity, power and influence would be generated and it would be possible to forge ahead with existing and new initiatives in nursing education, as well as incorporating some of the specific changes referred to earlier in this chapter. In this way effective nursing education could be provided which demonstrates its value by the improvements in the standards of care provided to patients and clients. Thus, the myth of nursing education as a luxury would be dispelled; it would be highly valued for its means of providing a 'different view' – a necessity for all who practise nursing.

REFERENCES

American Hospital Association (1979) Landmark Statement Consideration of Legislative Mandatory Continuing Education Proposals. *Journal of Continuing Education in Nursing*, **10**(5), Sep/Oct, 37–41.

Bendall, E.R.D. (1975) *So you passed nurse. An exploration of some of the assumptions on which written examinations are based.* Royal College of Nursing, London.

Commission on Nursing Education (1985) *The Education of Nurses: A New Dispensation*, Royal College of Nursing, London (Chairman: H. Judge).

Committee on Nursing (1972) *Report of the Committee on Nursing*, HMSO, London (Cmnd 5115), (Chairman A. Briggs).

Dodd, A.P.C. (1973) Towards an Understanding of Nursing. Unpublished PhD thesis, Goldsmiths College, University of London.

English National Board for Nursing, Midwifery and Health Visiting (1985) Professional Education/Training Courses: Consultation Paper. English National Board, London.

Fretwell, J.E. (1982) *Ward Teaching and Learning.* Royal College of Nursing, London.

Gott, M. (1948) *Learning Nursing*, Royal College of Nursing, London.

Hooper, J. (1985) Educators need to be more flexible. *Nursing Standard*, No. **384**, 14 Feb., 12.

Illinois NA page 14.

Ogier, M.E. (1981) Ward sisters and their influence upon nurse learners. *Nursing Times*, **77**, 2 Apr., Occasional Papers 41–73.

Pembrey, S. (1985) Project 2000: A framework for care. *Nursing Times and Nursing Mirror*, **81**, 11 Dec, 47–9.

Peters, R.S. (1965) Inaugural lecture – Education as initiation, in *Philosophical Analysis and Education* (ed. R.D. Archambault), Routledge and Kegan Paul, London.

Price Waterhouse (1987) *Price Waterhouse Report on the Costs, Benefits and Manpower Implications of Project 2000.* UKCC, London.

Statutory Instrument (1983) *The Nurses, Midwives and Health Visitors Rules Approval Order.* HMSO London (SI No. 873).

Statutory Instrument (1987) *The Nurses Midwives and Health Visitors (Entry to Training Requirement) Amendment Rules Approval Order.* HMSO, London (SI No. 446).

United Kingdom Central Council for Nursing, Midwifery and Health Visiting (1983) *Funding the Work of the UKCC : A Consultation Paper About Fees.* UKCC, London.

United Kingdom Central Council for Nursing, Midwifery and Health

Visiting. (1986) *Project 2000 – A New Preparation for Practice.* UKCC, London.

United Kingdom Central Council for Nursing, Midwifery and Health Visiting (1987) *Discussion Paper : Mandatory Periodic Refreshment for Nurses and Health Visitors.* UKCC, London.

White, R. (1985) Educational entry requirements for nurse registration : An historic perspective. *Journal of Advanced Nursing,* **10**(6) Nov, 583–90.

3 Theory to practice: implementation in the clinical setting

AUDREY MILLER

Ever since organized nursing began, nurses have been theorizing about nursing. At any time when ideas (concepts) are delineated, hunches developed by linking concepts together to help describe, explain, predict or prescribe nursing, and those hunches are then communicated and used in a number of situations, the beginnings of nursing theory are formulated (Meleis, 1985).

In Britain, early theories about nursing were communicated by Florence Nightingale in 1859. *Notes on Nursing* and *The Art of Nursing* were based on observations and experience of nursing practice and were focused on how nurses might provide care and comfort and on the environment in which care and comfort were provided. Nightingale described nursing as both an art and a science and her ideas provided the foundation of a knowledge base unique to nursing. After Nightingale, the emphasis moved from nursing to medical knowledge and ideas about nursing became focused on medical phenomena such as signs, symptoms, disease and medical and surgical procedures.

Many textbooks for nurses were written by doctors (Moroney, 1950; Toohey, 1953) and said more about medical specialties than about nursing care. Textbooks written by nurses also tended to focus on disease specialties, biological systems and nursing procedures and said very little about patients as human beings, or the significance of social or environmental factors in health or illness (Hector, 1960). Nursing practice became functionally orientated and practising nurses were busy with tasks and procedures and took little time to think, to reflect, or to question their own practice (Loomis, 1974).

During this period, nursing theory and nursing practice tended to separate, with one group of nurses involved in caring for patients and another group of nurses involved in teaching nursing. The term nursing theory was used to differentiate classroom teaching from ward practice and, as Bendall (1975), Hunt (1974) and Dodd (1973) demonstrated, there was a gap between the nursing theory taught in the classroom and the nursing which was practised in the wards. Ideas about how nursing ought to be practised diverged from how nursing was practised, and the practical knowledge of practising nurses came to be seen as of less value and relevance than the theoretical knowledge taught in schools of nursing (Bendall, 1975).

With the advent of university education for British nurses in the 1960s and 1970s, there was a growing interest in articulating, teaching and communicating nursing theory and increasing emphasis that nursing practice should become theory based. Nursing theory was now used to describe a set of interrelated ideas about nursing (Stevens, 1979) rather than a method of teaching nursing, and nurses began to question the existing knowledge base of nursing practice. McFarlane (1976) pointed to several studies of nursing practice which indicated that very little nursing practice was based on rational, scientific method and she said 'Our conventional wisdom stems largely from ritual and a medical model . . . a sound scientific basis for practice must be the aim of every nurse who wishes to lift the standard of nursing care from the mechanistic and ritualistic.'

Clark and Hockey (1979) also suggested that there was very little theoretical basis for much of the knowledge on which nursing practice was based. Other authors drew attention to the need for nursing to develop 'scientifically derived sets of understandings about patients and their needs which relate specifically to nursing concerns' (Aggleton and Chalmers, 1986b).

It seems that nurse theorists and nurse educators examined the knowledge base of present day nursing practice in Britain and found many gaps in that knowledge. They argue that the present day intuitive knowledge of practising nurses is of the wrong type, and should be replaced with empirically based, rational, scientific knowledge. In the view of nurse theorists, traditional 'know how' knowledge is no longer an adequate or valid basis for nursing practice and 'The time has come for knowledge validated by research to be the primary determinant of nursing practice' (Fawcett, 1980)

Authors also suggest that nursing theories (which are not usually research based) might be used to improve or change nursing practice.

> The most important task, however, will be for practising nurses to evaluate the appropriateness of each of these (nursing theories) against the demands of their own work situations. By doing so it may be possible to refine and develop the various approaches to nursing. (Aggleton and Chalmers, 1986a)

Thus it is argued that either through the application of knowledge validated by research, or through the application of knowledge articulated and communicated in nursing theories, or through the application of both of these, practising nurses might change and improve their nursing practices.

THE RELATIONSHIP BETWEEN THEORY, RESEARCH AND PRACTICE

Many authors stress that theory, research and practice should be closely related. As Jennings (1987) points out: 'Theory originates in practice and is refined by research. To be complete, theory must return to practice. In other words, practice serves as the origin for ideas for study, research is conducted to discover knowledge and theory is produced to guide practice.' The reality, however, seems to be that research, theory and practice are hardly related at all. The theoretical basis of nursing research is not strong (Brown, Tanner and Padrick, 1984) and the use of research to test theory is minimal (Silva, 1986). Research findings are not used in nursing practice (Hunt, 1981) and nursing theories are little used in nursing practice (Meleis, 1985). As Meleis (1985) said: 'Nurse theorists were developing theories in isolation, researchers pursued questions of interest only to educators and administrators and practitioners pursued their practices whilst oblivious to what the other two groups were doing.' This separation may have arisen because the type of knowledge which is valued by nurse theorists and nurse researchers is not seen as relevant by practising nurses, who use a different type of knowledge in their practice.

Philosophers, such as Kuhn (1970), observe that knowledge in an applied discipline such as nursing can consist of practical 'know how' knowledge which has evolved from decades of clinical experience and also 'know that' knowledge derived from theory. Kuhn points out that people have many skills (know how knowledge) and that people cannot always account for their know how. For instance, a nurse may lift a patient into bed, or comfort a crying child, or feed a patient with swallowing difficulties using know how knowledge and she may skilfully carry out these activities with, or without, theoretical knowledge about the mechanics of lifting or swallowing, or of the theory of child care. Theoretical 'know that' knowledge is the kind of knowledge which is developed in theories or models and contained in textbooks.

Burnard (1987) proposes, that in addition to intuitive 'know how' knowledge and theoretical 'know how' knowledge, personal knowledge and feelings may develop during the course of encounters and experience with people or things and he calls this 'experiential' knowledge.

If one accepts that these three types of knowledge are important in nursing practice, then knowledge development for nursing practice can consist of extension of theory based on empirical investigation of nursing practice and studies such as those of Hayward (1975) and Stockwell (1972) are useful. Knowledge development can also arise from investigation and charting of the existent 'know how' knowledge of practising nurses (Benner, 1984) and from investigation of personal actions within nursing practice (Clarke, 1986; Burnard, 1987).

APPLYING RESEARCH KNOWLEDGE INTO NURSING PRACTICE

The application of 'know that' knowledge may be seen to take place when nurses find reported research and apply it into their clinical practice. As long ago as 1972, the Briggs Report proposed that 'Nursing should become a research based profession' yet in

1981 Hunt pointed out that despite the availability of a certain amount of objectively determined factual knowledge which could provide practising nurses with indicators for practice, the use of research findings in clinical practice in Britain was minimal. She proposed that the reasons why nurses do not use research findings are that they do not know about them: they do not understand them; they do not believe them; they do not know how to apply them and they are not allowed to use them (Hunt, 1981). Greenwood, however, suggests that Hunt's views are simplistic and he argues that practising nurses do not apply research findings into their practice because they do not perceive them as relevant to practice. He says: 'Nursing is a practical activity, it is aimed at bringing about change in the physical, emotional and social status of persons – the problems that confront nurses are essentially practical problems concerning what to do.' He argues that nursing research has tended to approach nursing as though it were a theoretical activity and that situational, participatory action research which reveals to practitioners how theoretical abstractions relate to everyday practice is of more use in nursing practice than other types of research (Greenwood, 1984).

It is interesting to note that Greenwood's argument that nursing research should be based in nursing actions is part of a general move in nursing away from logical empiricism which emphasizes objectivity and strives to explain nursing through the testing of hypotheses and the development of theories. There is increasing recognition that nursing involves caring and nurturing activities within a social context and that attempts to investigate or to teach nursing using methods developed in the physical sciences are inappropriate. Many nurses suggest that it should be recognized that nursing is an art as well as a science and that nurses should value truths arrived at by intuition and introspection, as much as those arrived at by scientific methods (Silva, 1977).

Whether the different kind of nursing research advocated by Greenwood will be perceived as more relevant to practising nurses than that which already exists is open to question. Meleis (1985) suggests that knowing becomes knowing through a method of 'tenacity' in which people hold firmly to their beliefs due to psychological attachment to the thing they presume to know. In the case of nurses, knowing may arise from repeated clinical experiences and the nurse may refuse to modify her beliefs in the face of new evidence (Meleis, 1985). If this is so, then merely changing the way in which research is carried out will make no difference at all to whether practising nurses generally incorporate research findings into their clinical practice. It is more likely that knowledge of research findings introduced during, and closely related to, the nurse's repeated clinical experiences would facilitate attachment to that knowledge (and to that type of knowledge). For this to happen, the present focus of nurse education would have to shift so that the learner's personal experience and actions in the clinical area become the central focus of education, and educators would need to ensure that research-based knowledge is not only seen as a valuable adjunct to clinical practice, but that it becomes explicitly linked to concrete nursing actions within a particular clinical context. In this way, 'know that' knowledge would become a valued and integral part of the 'know how' skills developed in the course of practising nursing. Both Clarke (1986) and Burnard (1987) describe methods of achieving this and these will be discussed later.

NURSING THEORY AND NURSING PRACTICE

Meleis (1985) reviews the many definitions of nursing theory and points out that labels such as conceptual frameworks, conceptual models, paradigms, metatheories and perspectives have been used interchangeably to describe nursing theory. She argues that the different labels are different in emphasis rather than substance and that the use of a multiplicity of labels creates ambiguity and confusion, and produces time-wasting, non-productive argument about semantics. Meleis argues that the term 'nursing theory' can usefully replace all these different labels and it was decided that, rather than attempting to define and differentiate conceptual frameworks, models, paradigms and metatheories, the single term 'nursing theory' would be used throughout this chapter.

Meleis defines nursing theory as: 'An articulated and communicated conceptualization of invented or discovered reality in or pertaining to nursing for the purposes of describing, explaining, predicting or prescribing nursing care.'

Examination of Meleis' definition of nursing theory suggests that 'know that' theoretical knowledge of nursing has important

Table 3.1 The difference between 'know that' and 'know how' nursing knowledge

'Know that' theoretical knowledge	'Know how' practical and experiential knowledge
Articulated conceptualizations of nursing communicated in theories such as those of Orem (1971), Roy (1976), Rogers (1970) and Neuman (1980)	Often inarticulated conceptualizations of nursing – communicated by word of mouth and by role modelling
Based on invented or discovered reality	Based on personal experience in clinical practice
For the purpose of describing, explaining, predicting or prescribing nursing care	For the purpose of delivering nursing care to patients

differences from 'know how' nursing knowledge (Table 3.1).

The important question here is whether and how 'know that' theoretical knowledge can be useful in nursing practice, and to what extent 'know that' theoretical knowledge can or should be used to replace or to modify the 'know how' knowledge of practising nurses. In order to investigate this question, the potential benefits and problems of applying nursing theory into nursing practice in Britain will be discussed and some of the possible alternatives for knowledge development in nursing practice will be considered.

THE POTENTIAL BENEFITS OF APPLYING NURSING THEORY INTO NURSING PRACTICE

A great many of the potential benefits of nursing theory for nursing practice have been identified by nurse theorists.

Nursing theories offer a beginning articulation of what nursing is, and what roles nurses play. They offer a view of the underpinnings of nursing and they offer ways of how nurses can help patients. Theory provides the nurse with goals for assessment, diagnosis and intervention ... theory is a tool that renders practice more efficient and more effective ... theory helps to identify the focus, the means and the goals of practice. Using common theories enhances communications, increasing autonomy and accountability to care. Theory helps the user to gain control over subject matter. (Meleis, 1985)

Jacox (1974) points out that theories can be used not only to describe and explain nursing, but also to predict nursing situations with varying degrees of accuracy.

The many potential benefits and uses for nursing theory suggest that practice without theory will be ineffective and uninformed and there is no question that well-informed nursing practice is preferable to uninformed nursing practice and that effective nursing practice is preferable to ineffective nursing practice. How is it then, that despite the many potential benefits which nursing theory can offer nursing practice, the major uses of nursing theory so far have been in education rather than in practice or research? Meleis suggests that the sentiment of American nurse practitioners was to question the usefulness of nursing theory and to castigate nurse theorists for using esoteric language and for being far removed from the reality of nursing practice.

She argues that, because theories focused on education and professional identity, emergent theories were not used to guide practice or research but were used to guide teaching, and although theories may have indirectly influenced practice through students, they were little used by nurse practitioners (Meleis, 1985). Although Meleis is optimistic that theory and practice might now be more interrelated in America, the view of some American nurses suggests that continuing acquaintance with nursing theories has done little to bridge the gap between theory and practice and that both nurse educators and practising nurses felt that the nursing theories so far developed were useful frameworks for history taking and care planning, but offered little real guidance for nursing interventions (Webb, 1984).

It can be argued that a similar situation exists in Britain in the 1980s. When applied into nursing practice, nursing theory can provide a comprehensive framework and focus for assessing patients and for planning care but it is not easy to use the theory as guidelines or frameworks for nursing interventions. Despite an almost boundless faith in the potential benefits of nursing theory for nursing practice, its major utility so far appears to have been in nurse education. Perhaps this is because expectations of nursing theories and expectations of practising nurses are unrealistic, or perhaps it is because nursing theories which are useful for nursing practice have not yet been devised. As Walton (1986) points out,

> Models, like the nursing process and care plans before them, risk being seen as a panacea for all nursing's ills. Like the nursing process and care plans, they are expected to fulfil many different purposes simultaneously; to serve patient care needs by providing a comprehensive framework for their assessment, but also to further the professional academic desire to create a unique body of nursing theory and to delineate nursing's boundaries . . . Unrealistic expectations of models as of the nursing process, may be accompanied by unrealistic demands on practising nurses, requiring hard pressed staff with limited training opportunities to have theoretical knowledge of alternative models of nursing and the scientific information to practice the specific model chosen is a tall order.

THE UTILITY OF NURSING THEORY FOR NURSING PRACTICE

What does the practising nurse want or need from nursing theories? One can only speculate about this because the requirements of practising nurses do not seem to have been investigated. Although there is very little evidence that practising nurses are using nursing theory, this may be because the presently available theories are not relevant to nursing practice. It may also be because the theory of the nurse theorist is incongruent with the 'know how' knowledge of the practising nurse. Ogier and Barnett (1985) point out that the introduction of nursing process and other changes in nursing are already causing increases in the stresses of ward sisters and it seems unlikely that practising nurses would have the time, or the inclination to evaluate all the different nursing theories against the demands of their own work situations, as suggested by Aggleton and Chalmers (1986a).

However, if the practising nurse does want to choose a particular theory and apply it into practice, the utility of a theory for practice can be assessed by asking the following questions:

1. Does the theory have direct relevance for the way in which nursing is practised today in the British National Health Service?
2. Does the theory describe real or idealized 'ought to be' nursing practice?
3. Has the theory been tried and tested in practice situations/ have the assumptions and propositions of the theory been tested?
4. Does the theory include consideration of the environment in which nursing practice takes place and of the resource and contextual factors which influence nursing practice?
5. Is the theory applicable to the relevant area of nursing practice and does the theory fit in with the nursing process?
6. Does the theory provide enough direction to influence nursing interventions and does it predict the consequences of nursing interventions (i.e. is it prescriptive for nursing practice?)
7. Does the theory include concepts that are too abstract or too general to be easily applied to everyday practice – or concepts that are irrelevant to everyday practice?
8. Is the theory easy to understand? Are the concepts described in the usual language of practising nurses?
9. Is the theory congruent with, or widely different from, the 'know how' knowledge and the values of experienced nurses working in a particular area of practice?

DISCUSSION OF THE UTILITY OF NURSING THEORY FOR NURSING PRACTICE IN BRITAIN

Questions 1, 2 and 3

The utility of nursing theory for nursing practice is limited if the theory describes 'ought to be' practice which bears little relationship to real practice. These imagined ideas about nursing practice do not exist except in the mind of the nurse theorist who created them, and although they may provide useful perspectives for nurse education, their application and use in reality nursing practice is problematic. As Meleis (1985) says: 'Theirs was the vision of what nursing ought to be, of what care should be like . . . now we have the ideal goals, modifications of these theories will ensue as nurses begin to describe and document what is there and what is attainable.'

Although many nurse theorists state that nursing theory must arise and be closely related to nursing practice (Dickoff and James, 1975) some theories are abstract fantasies which are patiently unrelated to everyday nursing practice and impossible to apply in the context of care in which practising nurses work. The amount of testing in actual practice situations is very limited for some theories and Meleis' review of theories suggests that the more abstract and complex theories, such as those of Rogers (1970) have not been operationalized into practice. The theory most widely tested in practice is that of Orem (1971) and Meleis suggests that this is because Orem's theory incorporates the medical perspective and uses medical science language, and is developed around the ill person and institutional care.

The amount of research testing nursing theories has been extremely limited. A study of Silva (1986) indicated that, although very many nursing theories have been developed, only nine research studies have explicitly tested the validity of the assumptions and propositions contained in the various models during the past 30 years.

The advocates of nursing theory suggest the use of nursing theory will help to establish a scientific basis for nursing practice. It is noted, however, that many of the theories were devised for education and use ideas developed in other disciplines in order to describe idealized nursing rather than reality nursing practice. The assumptions and propositions contained in the theories are largely untested and it is not, perhaps, surprising that many theories have been little used in nursing practice. The main impetus for the use of nursing theory is from nurse educators, who use nursing theory as a framework for teaching and require learners to use a theoretical framework when they are learning how to assess patients and to plan care.

Questions 4, 5 and 6

Although most of the nursing theories devote a great deal of attention to the concept of the person and to the interaction between nurse and patient, the concept of the environment and the context of care are rarely mentioned. Kim (1983) and Meleis (1985) concur that there is a dearth of data regarding the environment. The only two theorists who have explored the importance of the environment are Nightingale (1859) and Rogers (1970). Although lack of attention to the environment is less important when theory is being used as an educational tool, resources, context and environment are tremendously important influences on the actual practice of nursing. Yet some theories use patient–nurse encounters as a central concept, and treat these encounters as though they occurred in a vacuum, rather than within the multiple constraints and influences of a particular context (King, 1971; Peplau, 1952; Orland, 1961). There is an implicit assumption in the literature that nursing practice will differ when different nursing theories are used and that the adoption of a nursing theory will result in improved nursing practice. There is no evidence that these assumptions are true, nor is there any evidence that the adoption of nursing theory can influence the constraints which operate within a particular nursing context. Yet the constraints of the context of care and the resources available are probably far more influential on how nurses practise nursing than any amount of nursing theory.

The neglect of the importance of the environment is a major problem for the use of most of the existing nursing theories as a framework for nursing practice. The two theories which do emphasize the importance of the environment (Nightingale, 1859; Rogers, 1970) are difficult to apply in nursing practice. Nightingale's ideas are useful but more than a century out of date and Rogers' ideas are largely incomprehensible and have not been fully operationalized.

Questions 7 and 8

The language used by nurse theorists can alienate practising nurses. Theorists often use obscure and complicated language, with frequent reference to psychological and sociological concepts which are unfamiliar to practising nurses. A great deal of theory has been written by American nurses who use English words differently from the British. One correspondent, in a letter to the

Nursing Times, commenting about an esoteric article on models of nursing, says:

> I suspect many of us cannot understand it . . . I am sceptical whether 'consideration of the supply of sustenal imperatives to the eliminative sub-system' will do much to alert the nurse of a particular patient's need for brown bread for breakfast, for example . . . Surely we can muster enough good sense and logic to construct workable systems of individualized care without wrapping them round in a cocoon of obscure language. (Wright, 1984)

As this nurse points out, much of what is written about nursing theory is so obscure that it is meaningless to the average nurse. Even when nurses are compelled to study theory – because they are 'doing a course' or undertaking some research – it is often difficult to understand and remote from their nursing experiences. Another problem is that many nursing theories are so all purpose, so all inclusive and so abstract that, in trying to explain everything, they explain nothing. As Dickoff and James (1975) said, 'some nurse theorists seem to be held captive by myths . . . of complete explicitness, of an absolute order of things'.

Many theories are so all inclusive and so abstract that it is difficult either to identify or extract the parts of the theory which might be useful for nursing practice and it seems that the gap between theory and practice is widening rather than reducing, and that the ever-growing number of unwieldy nursing theories provide barriers rather than bridges for knowledge development in nursing practice.

Question 9

The discussion so far has centred on the usefulness for practice of explicit nursing theories which use ideas borrowed from other disciplines and which were developed mainly for use in nursing education and it is argued that these theories have limited use for nursing practice because they are not based on reality nursing practice. They are largely context free and they are too abstract and unwieldy to be easily applied into practice. Many theories are also largely untested and untried in either research or practice.

However, the implicit theoretical basis which experienced

practising nurses use in every day nursing is equally, if not more, important than these 'imported' theories. Although these implicit practice theories have not yet been articulated and communicated, there is evidence that the theories do exist and that when they are brought to the surface, they take a very different form from the visions of the theorists who used theories developed for nurse education.

Work such as that of Benner (1984) demonstrates that different types of nursing knowledge underpin the actions of learner (novice) nurses and expert clinical nurses. Expert nurses operate using a 'Gestalt' where the nurse sees the situation as a whole, and using past concrete experiences as paradigms, she identifies the essentials and acts without considering irrelevant options. Her actions are usually context dependent and the expert nurse may have difficulty explaining why she acts as she does – except to say that she had an intuitive 'gut feeling' about the situation. Novice nurses rely on principles and context-free rules; they tend to see situations as a compilation of equally relevant bits and so have difficulty in identifying priorities. Just as when someone is learning to drive a car, performance is halting and the gears, brakes, accelerator, highway code and road conditions are all equally important. An expert driver can turn the car in a small space, and start or stop the car with his attention focused on road conditions. Use of the gear, brakes, accelerator and highway code are automatically incorporated into a smooth, skilled performance.

Benner's work has important implications for the application of nursing theory into nursing practice. She says:

> The linear ideal that theory must be generated first and then applied into nursing practice has given us a deficit view of nursing practice, allowing us to see only the gaps. We cannot afford to ignore knowledge gained from clinical experience by viewing it only from simplified models, or from idealized decontextualized views of practice. Nor can we afford to attend to and legitimize only what we learn from scientific experiments, the scope and complexity of our practice are too extensive for this.

Benner's study suggests that the application of nursing theories which are based on ideas developed to help learner nurses learn how to study nursing may actually obscure the 'know how' knowledge embedded in expert clinical practice. Nursing practice is relational and cannot be adequately described by theories that are context free and which do not include the content and function of nursing practice (Benner, 1984).

CONCLUSION – THEORY TO PRACTICE OR PRACTICE TO THEORY?

Nursing theories can be used as maps for those who lack experience in the clinical area. In this way, a nursing theory can serve as a guide through unknown territory and can substitute for lack of personal knowledge and experience. Nursing theories are essential teaching guides as they can spell out in detail what to do – for instance when used as a framework for assessment and care planning. However, theories can alienate nurses who have already developed clinical expertise. The theories are usually organized on the basis of the lowest common denominator and their use requires practising nurses to return to abstract principles and rules and the step by step details of problem solving and decision making which they no longer find useful. Proficient clinical nurses compare past concrete with current concrete whole experiences and act accordingly and this kind of holistic 'know how' knowledge and practice is hindered rather than helped by attempting to apply abstract principles and element by element context-free analysis. Gordon (1984) cautions that formal models have limited use for nursing practice and says, 'Let formal models in many cases be regarded as training wheels, essential for the first safe rides, unnecessary and limiting once replaced by greater skill. Let not reality be confused with the model. And let us not forget that the model is a tool, not a mirror.'

What then is the future for nursing theory in nursing practice? It seems that nursing theories are very useful educational tools which can be used to guide the practice of learner nurses who have limited knowledge and experience, and that they can provide useful frameworks for assessment and care planning. Other than this, their use in practice is of limited value. What is needed now is further work to surface, articulate and communicate the rich theory which underlies clinical practice and study of how this theory can be used to help learner nurses move more easily from being novices to becoming expert clinical nurses. Educators such as Burnard (1987) and Clarke (1986) approaching the problem from rather different viewpoints, and using rather different terminology, both suggest that the learner nurse's own nursing actions and experiences in the practice area should become the starting point for nurse education. Theory and knowledge can then be used to cause learners to reflect upon and discuss the rationale for their actions. Clarke (1986) says,

> The use of the psychology of personal action would, I believe anchor nursing theory within the reality of nursing practice. The keystone of theory would become the nursing action ... Nursing theories which developed out of a reflection on nursing actions would be middle range theories, couched in language acceptable to nurse practitioners, rather than all embracing theory couched in abstruse language. It follows that nursing research should centre on helping to elucidate the reasons for nursing action, the identification of the goals of nursing actions and in helping practising nurses in their choice of nursing actions.

Thus, it seems that practice to theory rather than theory to practice is now possible. Theory and research grounded in and closely applied to nursing practice has far better potential for improving the effectiveness and the knowledge base of nursing practice and for reducing gaps between theory, practice and research than theories generated outside practice and then applied to practice.

As Henderson (1987) in her ninetieth year had the wisdom to point out,

> When nurses' sensitivity to human needs (their intuition) is joined with the ability to find and use expert opinion, with the ability to find reported research and apply it to their practice, and when they themselves use the scientific method of investigation, there is no limit to the influence they might have on health care worldwide.

REFERENCES

Aggleton, P. and Chalmers, H. (1986a) *Nursing Models and the Nursing Process.* Macmillan, Basingstoke.

Aggleton, P. and Chalmers, H. (1986b) Nursing research, nursing theory and the nursing process. *Journal of Advanced Nursing,* **11**(2) Mar 197–202.

Bendall, E. (1975) *So you Passed, Nurse.* Royal College of Nursing, London.

Benner, P. (1984) *From Novice to Expert: Excellence and Power in Clinical Nursing Practice.* Addison-Wesley, Menlo Park.

Brown, J.S., Tanner, C.A. and Padrick, K.P. (1984) Nursing's search for scientific knowledge. *Nursing Research,* **33**(1) Jan/Feb, 26–32.

Burnard, P. (1987) Towards an epistemological basis for experiential learning in nurse education. *Journal of Advanced Nursing,* **12**(2) Mar, 189–93.

Clark, J.M. and Hockey, L. (1979) *Research for Nursing: a Guide for the Enquiring Nurse.* H.M. and M., Aylesbury.

Clarke, M. (1986) Action and reflection: practice and theory in nursing. *Journal of Advanced Nursing,* **11**(1) Jan, 3–11.

Dickoff, J. and James, P. (1975) Theory development in nursing, in *Nursing Research* (ed. P.J. Verhonick), Little, Brown, Boston.

Dodd, A.P. (1973) *Towards an Understanding of Nursing.* Unpublished PhD thesis, Goldsmith College, University of London.

Fawcett, J. (1980) A declaration of nursing independence: the relation of theory and research to nursing practice. *Journal of Nursing Administration,* **10**(6) June, 36–9.

Gordon, D.R. (1984) Research application – identifying the use and misuse of formal models in nursing practice, *From Novice to Expert: Excellence and Power in Clinical Nursing* (ed. P. Benner), Addison-Wesley, Menlo Park.

Greenwood, J. (1984) Nursing research: a position paper. *Journal of Advanced Nursing,* **9**(1) Jan, 77–82.

Hayward, J. (1975) *Information – a Prescription Against Pain.* Royal College of Nursing, London.

Hector, W. (1960) *Modern nursing: Theory and Practice.* Heinemann, London.

Henderson, V. (1987) *Clinical excellence in nursing – international networking.* Address to the Conference on Nursing Research, July 1987, Edinburgh.

Hunt, J. (1981) Indicators for nursing practice: the use of research findings. *Journal of Advanced Nursing,* **6**(3) May, 189–94.

Hunt, J.M. (1974) *The Teaching and Practice of Surgical Dressings in Three Hospitals.* Royal College of Nursing, London.

Jacox, A. (1974) Theory construction in nursing: an overview. *Nursing Research,* **23**(1) Jan/Feb 4–13.

Kim, H.S. (1983) *The Nature of Theoretical Thinking in Nursing.*

Appleton-Century-Crofts, Norwalk.

King, I.M. (1971) *Towards a Theory for Nursing*, Wiley, New York.

Kuhn, T.S. (1970) *The Structure of Scientific Revolutions*, 2nd edn, University of Chicago Press, Chicago.

Loomis, M.E. (1974) Collegiate nursing education: an ambivalent professionalism. *Journal of Nursing Education*, **13**(4) Nov, 39–48.

McFarlane, J.K. (1976) The role of research and the development of nursing theory. *Journal of Advanced Nursing*, **1**(6) Nov, 443–51.

Meleis, A. (1985) *Theoretical Nursing: Development and Progress.* Lippincott, Philadelphia.

Moroney, J. (1950) *Surgery for Nurses.* Livingstone, Edinburgh.

Neuman, B. (1980) The Betty Neuman health care systems model: a total person approach to patient problems in *Conceptual Models for Nursing Practice* (eds. J.P. Riehl and C. Roy), Appleton-Century-Croft, New York.

Nightingale, F. (1859) *Notes on Nursing – What it is and What it is not.* Harrison, London.

Nightingale, F. (1946) *The Art of Nursing.* Morris, London.

Ogier, M. and Barnett, D. (1985) Management: unhappy learners ahead? *Nursing Mirror*, **161**, 17 Jul, 18–20.

Orem, D. (1971) *Nursing: Concepts of Practice.* McGraw Hill, New York.

Orlando, I.J. (1961) *The Dynamic Nurse–Patient Relationship.* Putnam, New York.

Peplau, H.E. (1952) *Interpersonal Relations in Nursing*, Putnam, New York.

Rogers, M. (1970) *An Introduction to the Theoretical Basis of Nursing.* Davis, Philadelphia.

Roy, C. (1976) *Introduction to Nursing: An Adaptation Model*, Prentice-Hall, Englewood Cliffs.

Silva, M.C. (1977) Philosophy, science, theory: inter-relationships and implications for nursing research. *Image: The Journal of Nursing Scholarship*, **9**(3) Oct, 59–63.

Silva, M.C. (1986) Research testing nursing theory: state of the art. *Advances in Nursing Science*, **9**(1) Oct, 1–11.

Stevens, B.J. (1979) *Nursing Theory: Analysis, Application and Evaluation.* Little, Brown, Boston.

Stockwell, F. (1972) *The Unpopular Patient.* Royal College of Nursing, London.

Toohey, M. (1953) *Medicine for Nurses.* Livingstone, Edinburgh.

Walton, I. (1986) *The Nursing Process in Perspective: a Literature Review.* Department of Social Policy and Social Work, University of York, York.

Webb, C. (1984) On the eighth day God created the nursing process and nobody rested: *Senior Nurse*, **1**, 14 Nov 22–3, 25.

Wright, B. (1984) Abstract terminology. (Letter) *Nursing Times*, **80**, 10 Oct, 12.

BIBLIOGRAPHY

Jennings, B.M. (1987) Nursing theory development: success and challenges. *Journal of Advanced Nursing*, **12**(1) Jan, 63–9.
McFarlane, J.K. (1977) Developing a theory of nursing: the relation of theory to practice, education and research. *Journal of Advanced Nursing*, **2**(3) May 261–70.

4 Nursing management and leadership – the challenge

COLIN RALPH

This chapter will begin and end with the same message. The message is that all developments in nursing*, and indeed, all events in the world in which we live, should be judged against the climate and culture of their day. The development of nursing leadership is no exception. To judge developments and events without taking account of the broader social and health worlds of which nursing is a part is to see only one corner of a larger picture. So it is with the beginning of formal nursing leadership. The first notable nursing leader was Florence Nightingale but notable especially because of the prevailing climate and culture of her early pioneering days in the nineteeth century. The relevance of social class, the prevalence of disease – many now largely extinct in the Western World – and the position of women in society, all contributed to the circumstances of the day which made Nightingale such a lasting figure and symbol in the annals of nursing history.

Nightingale created a model for the organization of nursing and for institutional nursing leadership. Indeed, she set a striking precedent for participation in policy and administrative affairs.

---

*The word nursing is used to refer equally to midwifery and health visiting and nurse to refer equally to midwife and health visitor.

These factors were replicated by many hospital matrons over the years since Nightingale made her deep impression. These points are noted here not just for historical interest. They serve to underline the relevance of circumstances in society at large, which served to make Nightingale's contribution peculiar to the time and of such major significance.

In the years that followed Nightingale's development of what, in these modern days, we would probably call a framework for nursing management and leadership, a pattern emerged. Institutions – governed by boards and committees – appointed matrons to oversee the nursing and domestic services of their institutions, and many were responsible for nurse training. As years passed, laws changed, and the provision of health care became more organized and available and systems developed. Medical science, itself, developed and as medical treatment and care became more sophisticated so the nursing role changed and the content of the nursing curriculum expanded. All of these factors demonstrate the progressive evolution of the events in the world and the significant shift in our social and health profiles over the years.

During the First World War detachments of 'nurses' made a significant contribution to the care of the wounded. Many had no formal training, and some had varying degrees of preparation and experience, yet they came together from public, military and voluntary organizations to care for the sick and wounded. In the armed forces the nursing service grew between the Wars, and particularly after the Second World War, and was developed under the command of Matrons-in-Chief. In the public health field hospital matrons became key figures in hospital organizations. At the introduction of the National Health Service Act in 1948 nursing leadership, headed by its matrons and their assistants, stood ready to take its place in the new order of things.

During all of this time one point was consistent. The most senior nurse in the organization, usually known as the matron, whilst leading and managing her nurses, accounted for her actions and performance to another official. Such officials, over time, included superintendents, governors, secretaries of institutions, and in military services, medical officers. The nursing position in hospital, however, began to be more formally recognized within the National Health Service (NHS). In 1949 the King Edward's Hospital Fund for London opened the first of its Staff Colleges for

Ward Sister, followed in 1953 by a Staff College for Matrons. Regrettably, due to changing circumstances in the health services, they did not last long. In 1959 the Royal College of Nursing established a Working Party to study nursing administration. The result of the Working Party's endeavour was a number of recommendations for major changes in the traditional patterns of nursing administration.

The 1960s remain firmly fixed in the history of nursing management as the decade in which the *Report on Senior Nursing Staff Structure* (Salmon) was published. The Committee responsible for the report was chaired by Brian Salmon. Little did Salmon know that his work, and his association with the report, would be chronicled so firmly in the accounts of the profession's development. Since the time his report was published, Salmon must have found it difficult to imagine how misunderstood and misapplied his Committee's proposals were to be and how his name would become, particularly on the lips of doctors and even some nurses, a term used disparagingly to indicate bureaucratic systems that led to the best nurses being drawn away from clinical practice and in to posts in nursing management. More substantial accounts of the history of nursing should record the opportunity the Salmon Committee report created for the profession. Suffice to say here that the report recommended, and achieved, the establishment of nursing officer posts at each level of the National Health Service organization. For the first time in the life of hospital management committees, chief nursing officer posts were created at hospital 'group' level and replaced a varied set of arrangements that reflected the efforts of local hospital matrons to organize themselves to ensure that a nursing view was available at hospital management committee level and board of governor level in the case of teaching hospitals which was hitherto devoid of the presence of a nurse at this level of policy and management. The Salmon Committee proposals also linked highly stratified management principles to the organization of hospital nursing services and the distinction between first, middle and top management levels in nursing was made. This approach was so orderly that it was even possible to attach numerical significance to the place of senior nurses in the hospital nursing hierarchy.

The application of numbers in this way served only to discredit further the overall thrust of the report which was to place the previously unrecognized significance of nursing in a position, as of right, around all the decision-making tables of the organization. Calling nurses by number became commonplace and only led to the ridicule of the Salmon proposals as being managerially doctrinaire and inappropriate for British nursing. These factors apart, two further points must be recorded here. The first is that the profession itself was not allowed the advantage of awaiting the outcome of the Salmon pilot schemes designed to test the value of the Salmon proposals to the organization of hospital nursing, largely due to pressure for wholesale implementation, arising partly from the influence of the Prices and Incomes Board Report No. 60. These circumstances resulted in almost wholesale application of the recommendations which inevitably led to inappropriate application of the Salmon blueprint to the National Health Service.

The second point is that, had Salmon not reported when he did, it is unlikely that nursing posts at district and regional management team level in the 1970s, and district health authority level in the 1980s, would have been established. The Salmon recommendations pioneered these posts, and without them it is unlikely that these posts would have been created and the events that followed in the 1970s and 1980s would have been quite different.

It is the writer's hope that comprehensive histories of the profession will be more balanced in their assessment of the Salmon Report than its past and contemporary critics. The possibility for creating clinical posts above ward sister level, and for establishing a lasting place for top nursing leadership roles in the public health sector, together with an imaginative framework within which to structure nursing, was in the grip of the profession as a result of Salmon's proposals. For some, the temptation to rush toward a managerial model, without weighing the possible consequences of not considering its suitability for the effective development and management of clinical nursing practice and the creation of clinical roles, was too great. The adverse effect this had on the important relationship with the medical profession, on the fragile bridge between those who practised clinical nursing and those who managed them, cannot be over-emphasized.

Salmon was, nevertheless, here to stay, at least in some form or another until the early 1980s. So it was that the profession moved to the eighth decade of the century when its position was formalized still further, albeit temporarily, and, in theory at least, with an unprecedented model and position of authority for the management and leadership of the profession.

Similar trends were emerging in the community nursing services which at that time were part of local government services and not the national health service. The Mayston Report (DHSS, 1969) provided the community nursing equivalent of the Salmon proposals for the management and organization of hospital nursing services.

It had been apparent for some time that the management of community health services by local authorities, and of hospital services by the NHS, was inconsistent. During the late 1960s and early 1970s there was a prevailing view that it would be appropriate to integrate community and hospital-based services within the NHS. From a planning perspective such steps had great advantages as the health needs of communities and populations could be more readily viewed when managed by one agency. From the direct care perspective the advantage of the health service managing both hospital-based and community services had significant advantages. These included, not least, that of removing the organizational barrier between two agencies who were separately responsible for providing care for citizens who may cross the community and hospital boundary a number of times, for example, during any one episode of illness.

The word 'integration' became a key word in the NHS in the 1970s. The government, following the issue of green papers, decided that a reorganization of the health service to accommodate the integration of services was necessary. This decision reflected the general consensus within the service that such a step would be desirable and a White Paper was issued (Secretary of State for Social Services, 1972).

The steps taken to reorganize the health service were very well defined and the reorganization process across the country followed a very orderly pattern. Detailed arrangements for the management of the service were also set down in a published document which became known as the 'Grey Book'. Hospital management committees, and boards of governors in the case of teaching hospitals, stood down and newly created regional health authorities, area health authorities and district management teams were created. The style of management embodied in the 1974 reorganization of the NHS was that of consensus. Consensus management was achieved through organizational arrangements that ensured that key officers collaborated together at each managerial level charged with corporately managing the services for which they were responsible. Regional health authorities each had a regional team of officers consisting of a regional administrator, a regional treasurer, regional medical officer and regional nursing officer. Similarly, area health authorities also had an area team of officers consisting of senior personnel drawn from the administrative, financial, medical and nursing disciplines. Officers at regional and area levels were directly accountable to their authorities and many teams adopted the system of rotating chairmanship so that individual members chaired the team in turn. The majority of area health authorities were responsible for a number of health districts within their geographical area. Each health district was managed by a district management team and the teams consisted of a district administrator, district treasurer, district medical officer and district nursing officer. In addition district management teams were joined by a representative of general practitioners within the district, a representative of the consultant medical staff usually the chairman of the representative medical committee within the district and in districts where a medical and/or dental school was located, the Dean of the school was also a member of the team.

In the case of nursing, the functional management of nursing was retained by the district nursing officer. The district nursing officer was monitored by the area nursing officer and the relationship between district management teams and area teams of officers was one that caused some consternation and uncertainty. Whilst area health authorities were charged with managing health services throughout their area the individual health districts were managed by a team of officers who were accountable to the area health authority just as members of the area team of officers were. These district officers were monitored and coordinated, but not managed, by their area level counterparts. It would not be appropriate to dwell further on these organizational issues but they should be noted in passing especially as the relationship between areas and districts, in the newly built structures, later led to dissatisfaction with the new system. This was partly responsible for the elimination of area health authorities in the early 1980s and to which this chapter refers later.

In the development of nursing management and leadership the

1974 reorganization embodied all the aspirations of the profession at that time. Key nurses found themselves working collaboratively with their administrative, financial and medical colleagues as equal members of management or officer teams. Nurses at the three levels of the new 1974 reorganization (district, area and regional) took their place in the new corporate management of the NHS and this position seemed to embody all that the profession had long striven to achieve. This seemed a logical continuum to the developments from 1966 made possible by the introduction of the proposals of the Salmon Report. Salmon put in place key nurses to assume the new district, area and regional nursing roles within the new 'integrated' NHS.

The 1970s ended with integration and consensus being the buzz words of the decade within the health service. This discussion must be limited to considering the development of nursing management and leadership but the 1974 reorganization resulted in profound change. Medical officers of health, formerly part of the local government system, took their place as medical officers within the national health service. Community nursing services were managed by district nursing officers, usually through community nursing divisions, and one chief nurse managed both hospital and community nursing staff. Perhaps the most significant factor of all, apart from the organizational issues, was that for the first time since the inception of the NHS in 1946 one agency was charged with the responsibility for meeting the health needs of entire defined populations. The spirit of integration lived on well into the 1980s but the management style and structure did not. These were shortlived and as the eighth decade of the century drew to a close significant changes in the organization of the health service were but a year away.

The preceding and brief account of historical milestones in nursing management show a clear pattern from 1966. The Salmon and Mayston reports formalized the nursing organizational arrangements in hospital and community nursing services. Both reports strengthened the organizational position of nursing and prepared the ground for the position of nursing when the hospital and community services were integrated in the 1974 reorganization of the NHS.

Developments in the management of nursing in the 1980s, however, require special examination. From 1974 to 1981 there was a growing unease with the three tiers of NHS organization and management. The regional health authorities, area health authorities and district management teams were considered heavily bureaucratic and steps were taken by Government to streamline the organization. In 1981 a report was published that led to the abolition of area health authorities and health districts having their own health authorities instead. The report, 'Patients First' (Department of Health and Social Security and Welsh Office, 1979), was generally well received as it was seen to bring authority and decision-making closer to the level at which health care was actually delivered, that is at the district level. The report also satisfied the general desire, widely expressed within the service and outside, to eliminate one level of NHS management and streamline the system.

The nursing profession generally welcomed this change. The report gave birth to the notion of units of management and carried forward the established tradition of a tripartite management arrangement where an administrator, a nurse and a representative of medical staff would work together as a unit management team and manage units on a consensus management basis. This management style, of course, was not new to NHS staff. It was embodied in the detailed 'Grey Book' which set down management arrangements for the 1974 reorganization. The accountability of the unit team members remained essentially the same as it had since 1974. The unit administrator remained accountable to the district administrator and the unit nurse, who adopted the new title of director of nursing service which replaced the title divisional nursing officer remained accountable to the chief nursing officer at district level. Unit management teams often included finance officers and the medical members were generally, in the case of hospital units, the chairman of the representative medical committee. In the case of community units the medical member was usually an elected representative of general practitioners. The nursing position was not altered radically and the chief nursing officer retained her professional accountability to the new district health authority as had been the case with area nursing officers before the area tier of organization was removed by these changes.

The notion of the unit of management is worthy of further consideration before moving on. Nursing divisions, prior to 1981, were under the professional and managerial control of divisional nursing officers and were generally based on hospitals and community organizations that were smaller than the new units. The changes that stemmed from 'Patients First' generally reduced the number of divisions by grouping divisions in the new unit management arrangements. The grouping of divisions in this way created considerable debate and concern as larger units emerged. Some units grouped hospital and community services and mixed certain client-orientated services, for example elderly care services with acute hospital services and community services with priority care services. Many nurses, doctors and others were fearful that the progress made in developing services for the elderly, mentally ill and handicapped, and in primary care services, would be lost and these services may become overshadowed by the generally larger and more costly acute hospital divisions with which they were being attached. The concern with size also led some to suggest that large units would lead to sub-unit systems of management being established and yet another tier of management creeping into the new system, albeit at a different level, but nevertheless distancing the unit management team from the services they were charged to manage.

These changes created great opportunities for the nursing profession to examine the nursing structure and to look again at nursing management processes. There had been a degree of disenchantment with the previous model, based on the Salmon recommendations. The profession, and indeed the medical profession, considered that nurses had still not got it right and many doctors were hostile to the nursing officer roles. Many chief nurses and directors of nursing service took the opportunity to introduce new structures with a swing away from conventional nursing officer posts to more clinically related posts that combined managerial responsibility with specialist clinical functions. Grading indication factors were developed for director of nursing service posts, and factors for examining the managerial and clinical components of nursing management posts at middle level devised. These events had two particularly interesting consequences. The first was that the grading factors for director of nursing service posts resulted in directors being assimilated to pay scales which were largely comparable with their administrative counterparts and, indeed, in some cases the nurse on the unit management team received a higher salary than her administrative team colleague. This development was quite unlike the historical trend of nurses generally earning less than those in the administrative discipline. The second was that there was a general shift away from service to managing discrete clinical areas or services. In some cases nursing officers became clinically based, taking the role and style of senior sister, with a coordinating and managerial role in relation to other wards or services. These innovations were, and are, deserving of greater attention and evaluation and may set new role models for the future.

The beginning of the 1980s represented a time of great change for the service and marked just the beginning of continuing change well into the decade. The period of adjustment to the new health service structure took time and although the process began in 1981 some districts had not filled key posts in the unit structures until well into 1983, and some still later. District health authorities had to be created and key appointments made at district level. The officers then recommended the organization of units to their authorities and these proposals were often the subject of detailed consultation and debate. The next step, when the configuration of units was known, was the appointment of unit management teams who, in turn, considered their organizational needs and the structures required to manage the units. These events also took time and some unit management teams remained incomplete for long periods. The teams and the service were to face further change. The change that was to follow was more radical and far-reaching than any the service had experienced or than many could have imagined. The story of this further change begins in 1983.

During the second term of the Conservative Government there was a general concern to tighten accountability and to consider the cost-effectiveness of services and their results. There was also, both within the service and outside the NHS, discontent with the consensus style of management. A number of studies had revealed flaws in this style which suggested that in some cases decision-making was unnecessarily protracted, that compromise solutions were often the outcome of debate as differing and conflicting interests had to be satisfied within the teams (both at unit and district levels), and that this method of management was cumbersome and that no one individual was clearly in charge.

These were some of the factors which led to the Secretary of State for Social Services to commission an inquiry into the management of the National Health Service. The approach to this inquiry was new. Previous reorganizations had been influenced by committees and the reports they produced. On this occasion the Secretary of State asked a team of three men from industry to conduct the review and report their findings to him. The inquiry team was led by Roy Griffiths, the Managing Director of a large company, who was later to become Deputy Chairman of the NHS Management Board which was created as a result of one of the inquiry team's proposals. The approach and style of the team's report was also new. Griffiths wrote a long letter to the Secretary of State setting out his proposals and although the report was in the form of a letter of some 24 pages it has since become known as the 'Griffiths Report'. The effects of the introduction of the proposals have been profound and it is necessary to restrict the debate to those proposals which have had particular implications for the profession and for the service. A great deal has been written about the report and its consequences, and it is unnecessary to repeat it here, particularly as a large proportion of what has been written concerns structural organizational matters which were but a part of the range of recommendations the inquiry team made to the Secretary of State. Of rather more importance, in developing an understanding of the consequences for the profession, is the social and political climate that prevailed at that time. The recommendations of the Griffiths report, then, should not be seen as only being relevant to the health service and a pre-occupation with how it is managed. The proposals reflected trends in society at large and the report was consistent with political beliefs and trends of the day.

The most significant proposal for the profession was the recommendation that general managers should be appointed at all levels of the service. Following acceptance of the proposals by the Secretary of State general managers were appointed at regional, district and unit levels in the service. The days of consensus management, as the service had known it, came to an end. So did the established pattern of control of nursing by nurses, formalized in the 1960s by the Salmon and Mayston proposals, and cherished by the profession. The response to the proposal to appoint general managers was predictably fierce from the profession. Many saw this new style of management as sweeping aside the control of the profession which was itself only recently secured and for which the profession had fought long and hard. The appointment of general managers was seen to threaten the power-base that the profession had enjoyed for 17 years through automatic membership of unit, district and regional management teams and their equivalents and through the professional and managerial control of nursing services and nursing education. The report did, however, acknowledge the importance of nursing leadership and nursing advice and when the profession recovered from the initial blow it turned its mind to translating the importance of these notions of leadership and advice to organizational reality.

The Government made it clear that the new general manager posts were open to able managers from all professions and disciplines. Nurses were encouraged to apply but both the level of applications, and successful appointment of nurses, remained low in the early stages. For the profession there were a number of serious concerns. These included the loss of the consensus management style and a real anxiety about the role of nurses at policy and management level. A second concern was preserving access to health authorities on professional matters, and a third was the challenge to conventional nursing management arrangements within units. At district level the profession saw the loss of the title, and often the post, of chief nursing officer and at unit level the title and post of director of nursing service. In some units the nursing officer or senior nursing manager role was also changed and unit general managers began to reshape the unit structures and align management structures with services such as in-patient and out-patient services or by specialty. Sub-units of management also began to emerge in which sub-unit general managers managed geographical or client-based services. These developments often blurred the position of nurses at both middle and more senior levels of management even more.

All these events caused great dismay within the profession. This culminated in a major campaign, launched by the Royal College of Nursing, to draw the attention of the public and politicians to the effects of the introduction of general management on the nursing profession. Questions in the House of Commons and debates in both Houses of Parliament ensued, together with high level meetings between leaders of the profession and Ministers in an attempt to safeguard the position of the profession in these changes. There was, inevitably, a considerable degree of acrimony but a number of letters of guidance to health authorities were issued by the Department of Health to clarify the professional role of nurses within the new management arrangements (Hansard, 1986a,b)

All these changes posed a new and unprecedented challenge to the profession. Nurses were required to articulate their special role and contribution to policy and management as nurses and not only as managers. The influence of professional participation in the management process was under examination and some general managers believed that membership of management groups, simply because professionals had been there before, or because nursing represented such a large percentage of the NHS work-force, was just not good enough to justify such positions. Many key nurses themselves, who for some years had been part of consensus management groups, and who were required to participate in that forum as members of 'corporate' teams, were suddenly in a position of explaining the discrete nursing contribution they bring to management. The years following 1983 were difficult ones for the profession and its leaders. A degree of disillusionment with conventional nursing management also began to emerge from within the profession and from others who had the opportunity to scrutinize the profession closely for the first time as a result of these changes.

But the changes also created new opportunities. The introduction of general management caused staff to examine the nature of the service and their responsibilities very carefully. The particular question of the provision of nursing advice to health authorities and management and leadership posed new, but potentially influential, and positive challenges.

To consider the effects of the introduction of general management to the NHS alone can lead to the belief that these changes were peculiar to the health services. They were not. Government had been concerned to improve the cost-effectiveness and efficiency of a number of state services and to tighten accountability. In this sense the process had been a success within the service and the special challenge to the profession has been to adjust to the management of the service. For the purposes of this chapter, in chronicling the development of nursing management and leadership, these changes can be seen to be profound and at first a threat but also a new challenge to the profession.

Before looking to the future, another significant event of the 1980s deserves special mention here. This is an issue of a series of proposals for the reform of nursing education.

As a result of proposals presented by the UKCC and National Boards (see Chapter 2), in March 1987 Ministers wrote a detailed letter to the service asking for responses to specific questions. The questions related to the proposals for educational reform and to the manpower and financial consequences for health authorities and managers. The service was also consulted on proposals for the introduction of a new support worker to assist the nurse, midwife and health visitor in her work. This process occurred at a time when nursing was already a high profile subject for a number of important reasons that should be stated at this stage.

The first of these was the focus on nursing manpower and the cost-effectiveness of nursing service and skill mix. The Comptroller and Auditor General, in his report to Government in 1985, recommended steps to improve the management of nursing manpower and for the service to develop more sophisticated systems for determining nursing manpower requirements. The second reason for this focus was the predicted reduction in 18-year-old females entering the employment market in the 1990s due to a fall in the birthrate in the 1970s. It is from this group of the population that nursing has traditionally recruited large numbers of student and pupil nurses. Indeed, during the third and fourth quarters of the 1980s some schools of nursing were already experiencing a reduction in the number of entrants to nurse training and a fall in recruitment of trained nurses to some areas. The expectation of increasing difficulties in recruiting, and concern about the loss of students during training and trained nurses from the service, highlighted by the Project 2000 Report, ensured that the health service looked critically and closely at the proposals for the reform of nursing education.

In order to assist health authorities to predict the possible financial and manpower consequences of the Project 2000 proposals the UKCC developed, in association with a firm of management consultants, a manpower model for the use of health authorities. The model required the manpower information, including wastage, retention and other factors, to be computed and allowed authorities who chose to use the model to look at the local impact of varying some of these factors, and particularly those relating to retention and wastage. There were a number of difficulties associated with this model and it was not well received in some areas. Despite the problems, and inevitable criticisms, it enabled health authorities to focus on nursing manpower in a way that many had not done before. The information on nursing manpower required to test the model was not easily obtained in some areas but in all places it placed nursing manpower centre stage and under scrutiny.

It would not be appropriate to pursue further the content of Project 2000 here, or the specific and very interesting question of nursing manpower. These matters, however, are extremely relevant to the unfolding story of nursing management. Nursing became a high profile matter within the health service within a short time of general management being established. The proposals for educational reform, and their possible consequences, resulted in the exposure of the profession in a way not experienced before. The profession, prompted by the Project 2000 Report and the debates that followed, revealed details of current practices, methods of training, and the anomalies and problems with the current system. The profession publicly declared its dissatisfaction with the current arrangements and supported the proposed remedies and improvements. In addition, and somewhat ironically, these practices brought nursing management and its practices under very critical examination and, in particular, its management and personnel practices were related to retention and recruitment rates which had been identified by the application of the manpower model and by health authorities. 'Non-nurses', for the first time, were invited to wander through the corridors of nursing and to look into previously dimly lit areas of nursing practice, education and management. In some corridors very rudimentary and inadequate nursing manpower information systems were to be found or, rather more precisely, were found to be missing.

During ministerial consultation on Project 2000 the profession has shared its circumstances and systems with the health service at large and a greater degree of understanding has been achieved. It is also significant to note that there was a general acknowledgement that reform of nursing education is needed if the profession is to be placed on a more satisfactory and robust footing for the future. One final comment must be made on the Project 2000 proposals. It is not unknown for professions to be criticized for being concerned with self-interest rather than the interests of those they exist to service (see Chapter 1). The Project 2000 Report is a pertinent example of how wrong such generalizations can be. The opening chapters draw heavily on the changing health needs of society, the shift from institutional to community care and the need to produce a flexible and able practitioner for the future, whose preparation is influenced by contemporary health needs and policy, and by service direction. It is on questions such as these that they report proposed change for the future in order to ensure that society receives a high standard of care from its nursing profession. Project 2000 – the process and the debate – indicated a new emphasis on the use of manpower information as an integral part of policy decisions. The Government consultation process, using both specific questions and the manpower model, heralded a new approach to management from the centre and new challenges for the management of nursing. These will be considered in the concluding part of this chapter.

NURSING LEADERSHIP AND ADVICE

From 1983 general management was quickly introduced to the service and appointments made at regional, district and unit levels. By 1986 there was a regional nursing adviser to all of the 14 regional health authorities in England and, although many had additional responsibilities to the provision of nursing advice, their primary function was the provision of nursing advice to authorities and to managers. At district level most health authorities had, by this time, appointed a nurse charged with the task of providing the health authority and its managers with informed and quality nursing advice. A range of titles of these posts have emerged in the service, and the range of post titles varied across all posts and all disciplines.

In some cases the nurse in this position was appointed on a full-time basis to advise on nursing matters and to lead the profession within the district. Many chief nurses were also responsible for other management functions and were often required to accept responsibility for quality assurance within the district. In a large number of cases the incumbent chief nursing officer was appointed to the new nursing post at district and regional level, and in a few cases new approaches were tried. These included the option of a director of nursing service within a unit of management, or a director of nursing education, acting as chief nursing adviser to the district health authority. These various models have been the subject of research and studies commissioned by the North West Thames Regional Health Authority and the Nursing Policy Studies Centre at the University of Warwick have examined the impact of general management on nursing. The effects on nursing, and of the nursing contribution to the management and policy process, deserve further study and evaluation.

Weaving the strands of these events together creates quite a different tapestry for nursing management and leadership by the end of 1988 from the picture at the beginning of that decade. Although at each level of management a senior nursing post exists to provide advice and leadership, the management function of nursing at district level had gone. Nursing and managerial minds focused on the nature of advice and leadership and its distinction from traditional nursing management roles, which had combined professional and managerial responsibility for nursing in a clear hierarchical pattern linking nurses in a line-management relationship. The well-established pattern gave way to nurses at unit, district and regional levels becoming managerially account-able to general managers and, at district and regional levels in particular, dual accountability – to general managers for manager-ial functions and to health authorities for professional functions – emerged. The maintenance of this latter relationship to health authorities was hard fought by the professional organizations for doctors and nurses. Similarly, at unit level, unit nurses were managerially accountable to unit general managers and profession-ally accountable to the chief nursing adviser to the health author-ity. These arrangements created both controversy and opportunity, and served to rekindle the interest in professional advisory committees for nursing and midwifery at district and regional levels. This interest warrants further discussion before considering other events at that time.

In 1974, area and regional health authorities were required to establish nursing and midwifery advisory committees and this was done with varying degrees of enthusiasm and success throughout the service. At the time of restructuring the service in 1981, health authorities had the option of creating these committees and some districts did not rush to set them up. The earlier committees had excluded the district nursing officers from membership at area committee level and were generally not well received as additions to the professional nursing network in some areas. The luke-warm response to the opportunity of establishing similar committees again in 1981 stemmed from the general dissatisfaction with the earlier experience from 1974. It is remarkable that these committees did not receive detailed attention and study for they created a historical precedent for the profession. For the first time a platform was established for nurses from clinical practice, education and management to come together to consider professional matters at health authority level. The committee membership comprised nurses who had not, hitherto, had the opportunity of contributing to policy discussions on professional matters or the experience of meeting together with the most senior nurse at area or regional health authority levels. They also, most significantly of all, created a formal link between the nursing committees and the health authorities. Apart from one study in particular the committees were not evaluated and generally lost favour over the years since their inception in 1974.

It is possible to contemplate that if the experience of these committees had been more positive the impact of general management on nursing from 1983 would not have been so profound. Embodied in these committees, and their constitutions, was the belief that the considered advice of nurses, midwives and health visitors – and not just the most senior nurses in the organization – was of value. The advisory committee machinery was extended to nursing as it had been to medicine and other professions who established comparable committee arrangements at the same levels of the health service organization. It could be argued that the lack of success with these nursing committees was the result of committee members being unable to see the breadth of the issues they were considering at this level and the lack of individual influence of members or the committee generally as a result of the ways the committees were structured.

The provision of nursing advice will be discussed in the last section of this chapter but it must be stated here that the profession, between 1974 and 1981, had in its grasp a model of committee structures that transcended the traditional nursing management hierarchy and provided a new and unprecedented opportunity for nursing. Their failure was, in part, caused by strict adherence to hierarchical principles which generated negative attitudes to the committees within the profession itself and which often crippled their potential for success. There were, of course, other reasons for the advisory committees failing generally in their task. The stark fact remains, however, that the opportunity was missed and the price was to be paid in the mid-1980s when the profession struggled to demonstrate to general managers and health authorities the importance of informed nursing advice and the nursing perspective in the policy and decision-making process. Interestingly, and almost as testimony to this argument, a new enthusiasm for creating professional advisory committees and networks at district level quickly emerged at this time. These steps indicated an attempt to 'regroup the troops' following the foray into general management. They also indicated a belated acknowledgement that for top nurses to be able to fulfil their responsibilities to provide nursing advice to health authorities and their managers they must be informed. They must also enjoy the support of their more junior professional colleagues throughout the district, whom they no longer manage.

All of these factors – the introduction of general management, the proposals for the reform of nursing education, demographic predictions, the scrutiny of nursing manpower, concerns for future recruitment and retention of nursing staff – placed nursing at the top of many managerial agendas. Together they posed nursing and the health services with pressing and serious questions and problems. The basis of staffing levels, the methods of predicting manpower requirements and the link between grade and skill mix in clinical settings and outcomes of care required answers. In many cases work had been completed to set a rational basis for staffing patterns but in others the patterns were largely historical. The debate on grade and skill mix, which is likely to continue to occupy the minds of the professions and managers for many years, has required nurses to articulate the connection between levels and ratios of nursing levels and qualifications to the nature and standard of care required. At the same time events in the public sector generally, and in particular the employment and manpower position in society in the 1980s, have influenced debates and the shape of events yet to emerge fully.

THE FUTURE AND THE CHALLENGE

This chapter began with an account of developments in nursing management and leadership and particularly focused on events from the 1950s. Inevitably this is not exhaustive and it is written, quite deliberately, from a nursing perspective for this is required in the context of this book. The account has tried to connect events and issues faced by nursing management and leadership and a number of these will be pursued further in drawing this chapter to a close and in looking to the future.

Society in the 1980s is now more sophisticated and medicine and health care has advanced beyond recognition. The organization of the National Health Service has changed significantly since its introduction in 1948. So, too, has the profession. It has developed and evolved as advances in medicine and health needs of society has progressed and changed. The curriculum for nursing preparation has been expanded and modified to reflect the new and developing roles of nurses in clinical practice and the aspirations of the profession itself. For nursing managers and leaders, the last decade has seen an unprecedented time of change and the culture of the service has shifted from a professionally led NHS to a managed service. These general descriptions indicate great change. Although the professional power-base of nursing, and other professions, can be seen to have changed as a result of the loss of the managerial stronghold of self-management by the professions, the need for a form of consensus remains. Consensus management may have given way to general management but it is inevitable that within a complex multi-professional service, such as the health service, a high degree of organizational co-operation and consent is necessary for the effective function of the organization. This is not to suggest, for one moment, that any profession has, or should have, the potential to sabotage the mechanics of the system. It does, however, point to the need to recognize and allow the expression of the professional ethic in the organization and management of the health service. The position of the profession within the health service, and the special contribution of nursing to health care, offers a suitable starting point for considering the future challenge to nursing management and leadership.

Despite organizational change the nursing service has been, and will continue to be, concerned with the provision of direct and safe care to patients and clients. The service exists to treat and care for citizens who fall ill and who require skilled care and to promote health. The range of need and provision is vast and can extend from a demented old man in a long-stay institution to a young woman in labour. Nurses, midwives and health visitors engaged in direct care are registered with the profession's statutory regulatory body, the UKCC, and are required to observe the Council's Code of Professional Conduct. The values of the profession, and the Code, together with the ethics that are inherent in professional practice, place the supremacy of patients above all things. The professional is required to serve the interests of those in his or her care and to take all steps to ensure standards are maintained and the integrity of the individual is respected. It is in this arena that questions of standards of patient care and safety place the health service in a special position in relation to other organizations and managerial models. The profession enjoys a special relationship with society and exists to serve those in need of care. It recognizes the vulnerable position of citizens when their health, for whatever reason, is impaired.

The profession faces a special challenge to articulate the effects of manpower, financial and managerial initiatives on standards of care. If general managers place great importance on delivering high standard services to patients, as they do, it is necessary for them to ensure that the organizational arrangements reflect the position and contribution of the professions. This must allow issues relating to standards of care and patient safety full and appropriately free expression within the organization. This is not to suggest that these matters are outside the general management system or structure. It is, rather, to suggest that nurses must be able to express the nursing practice position at all levels of decision-making, not merely for professional self-interest, but because managerial systems must take account of the consequences for patients in their decision-making. Nursing managers need new networks to ensure that these matters are identified and analysed and communicated to the appropriate levels and articulated in a form that conveys concrete and quantified messages and measures to managers and to health authorities. These networks include advisory arrangements that involve clinical nurses, to harness their valuable and essential contribution, and improve the quality of advice received by health authorities and managers. The days of rhetoric have gone. The new age of considered and costed decisions, both in terms of effectiveness and benefits, is here and here to stay. In order to fulfil this function properly nursing managers will require both professional and managerial development to prepare them fully for this task.

The accountability of the nurses to their professional regulatory body, the UKCC, and of course to their own conscience and to the law, can be described as professional accountability. It is suggested that professional accountability in nursing can be defined as that obligation on the nurse which binds him or her to a code of conduct. This is based on the expectations of society that the person will use discretion and skill to safeguard patients and act in every way to uphold professional standards. This obligation and the values of the profession, provide a framework for professional and ethical behaviour with which nurses must personally and professionally conduct themselves and within the primacy and vulnerability of those served is observed. This should not be considered to conflict with managerial accountability and the values of the profession should be seen to enhance the quality and sensitivity of the management of the service. Indeed, the existence of the Code of Conduct can positively assist nurses in taking steps to improve standards and work in the interests of patients and the service. It will be necessary for the profession and its leaders to continue to share its beliefs and values with others and to ensure that full account is taken of professional values whilst recognizing and accepting new managerial challenge.

The management of nursing manpower, and the cost-effectiveness of nursing care, will continue to pose special requirements on the profession and its managers. It is simply not enough, in this age and in the future, to say that all patients require skilled nursing care by qualified nurses. The manpower predictions, both as a result of the fall in the birth rate in the 1970s, and the inevitable competition among professions and employers for the more able recruits from the population, will require particular attention. For these reasons, and for those of cost, an intense interest in the levels of qualification and skill needed to deliver nursing care exists and will increase. So, too, will the emphasis on outcomes of nursing and indicators of performance.

The health world, and almost all that happens within it, is a reflection of events in the broader political and social worlds of which the health world, and the nursing profession, is a part. The recent emphasis on costs, outcomes, monetary and other values, will continue and nursing managers will increasingly be required to articulate arguments and proposals in economic as well as professional terms. Merely perpetuating historical trends will not be enough and the reference in this chapter to nursing manpower indicates the trends the profession should be prepared to expect. To meet this challenge effectively calls for nurses in management to be fully prepared for the nature of their roles. It also calls for foundation and post-qualification nursing curricula to reflect these changing demands on the role of the nurse, midwife and health visitor. The demographic predictions will call increasingly on nursing management to demonstrate that its personnel and management practices are flexible and imaginative so that recruitment and its techniques are maintained and improved so that staff are retained. The changing population trends are likely to lead to increased part-time appointments, improved child-care facilities for the children of professionals and to the introduction of local incentives to retain staff.

The ability of nursing management to recruit and retain staff will be a crucial challenge. The requirement concurrently to demonstrate cost-effectiveness of nursing care will increase. Conventional grade mixes in nursing teams was under scrutiny in the 1980s and this will continue as both the supply of trained nurses decreases and steps to improve the performance of the service and reduce operating costs increase. Nursing leaders and managers will be required to apply and refine tools that relate quality of care to costs and articulate the results in quantified and qualified terms.

These challenges to nursing management and leadership will be posed within a general management context. The introduction of general management to the National Health Service was difficult for the profession but the style will remain for some time. The challenge both for general managers and for the profession is to find a way of successfully interweaving professional advice and leadership within a general management system. General managers must enable this to happen and recognize the importance of effective nursing advice and leadership to the general management process. It is for the profession, however, to demonstrate that this can work and that it can enhance and contribute to the policy and management of the service. For this to be achieved nursing management must be committed to participating in a meaningful way. This requires mutual recognition and trust. General management must work for the good of the service and quality nursing leadership and management is integral to the effective general management of the service as a whole.

The management process itself will become more sophisticated. Improved financial systems, the application of information technology and experimentation with alternative methods of funding health services are all likely to increase. Nursing should, and indeed must, identify able leaders and managers to assume general management posts in the health services and to work with others in shaping new systems and policies. It is only through positive and full collaboration with managers and authorities that the values of the profession can continue to be carried forward and cherished through changing systems and cultures. This is not simply for the sake of tradition alone. As the concentration on performance and results intensifies, so the concern of the profession with the position of the individual in need of care becomes even more imperative.

For these challenges to be met the profession has to acknowledge that a number of internal steps are needed. The first of these is the construction of new bridges between nurses who practise nursing and nurses who manage nursing. For nursing leadership to really work leaders must have the support of clinical nurses and must be seen to be concerned with clinical issues and with improving standards of practice and care. A nursing manager who relates to clinical nurses in terms of cost-effectiveness and managerial issues alone, using managerial language, is unlikely to be a credible leader among clinical nurses. Similarly, a nursing manager who only relates to general managers in managerial terms, and who fails to articulate the professional dimension of care and standards, is unlikely to demonstrate the need for nursing, rather than general, managers in key managerial posts which include responsibility for nursing service. Conversely, a nursing manager who only communicates the professional perspective without due regard to managerial, financial and other considerations, is hardly likely to make a penetrating contribution to management. This discussion illustrates the complexity of the issues involved. The management of nursing requires a balance between concerns for safe and desirable standards of clinical practice and effective management. The challenge to nursing managers is to keep both responsibilities always in a degree of equilibrium so that the clinical and practice-related issues are given the clear leadership and attention they deserve. They must be balanced with prevailing managerial requirements and an astute sense of the requirements of the management system. Maintenance of such an equilibrium will give the profession the position and the leadership it requires and secure a meaningful place for the profession in the general management system.

The second step is the appropriate preparation of nursing, midwifery and health visiting staff. This is not just a question of providing management development opportunities for senior staff. Initiatives are required at all levels. The proposals for the reform of nursing education provide a new foundation for preparation for practice which reflects changing health care needs and health policy. The profession continues to struggle to achieve a structure for clinical practice but whatever the outcome of this endeavour measures are needed to retain skilled nurses in clinical practice and to identify those who aspire to enter nursing education and nursing and general management. The traditional method of allowing selected nurses to gravitate upwards through the nursing hierarchy in an orderly fashion, spending 'acceptable' periods of time in each post, has no place in the new order of things. The structures have changed but, more importantly, the profession must continue to identify and encourage those with exceptional ability at an early stage, and actively assist them to progress to key leadership positions in all areas of the profession and, indeed, in general management.

The third step is the profession's relationship with the medical profession. Nursing and medicine have much in common and share a similar value system that underpins professional practice. Doctors and nurses are the key players in the field of treatment and care. The complementary nature of nursing to medicine, and the importance of collaboration with medicine in developing the nursing profession itself, must be recognized if initiatives are to succeed. As the manpower position worsens, and as questions of maintaining minimum safety and standards displace less pressing matters at the top of key agendas, the joint co-operation between doctors and nurses will be essential for maintaining standards for those in need of care.

The fourth and final step suggested here is the need for the profession to acknowledge that the process of change will continue. For the profession to continue to adjust, flexibility in thought and a swiftness to adapt are necessary if the profession is to move forwards in a positive and developmental way. All of the issues identified in this chapter call for multiple nursing strategies that are sensitive to the broader issues and changes that shape our professional lives and our destiny.

BIBLIOGRAPHY

Clay, T. (1976) *The role of nursing and midwifery advisory committees in the reorganised NHS.* Unpublished MPhil thesis, Department of Government Studies, Brunel University.

Committee of Public Accounts (1986) *Fourteenth report: control of nursing manpower: Department of Health and Social Security, Scottish Home and Health Department and Welsh Office session 1985–86.* HMSO, London.

Davies, R. and Farrell, C. (1980) *Conflict and Consensus: an Analysis of the Evidence Submitted to the Royal Commission on the National Health Service 1976–1979.* King's Fund Centre, London (KF project paper RC1).

Department of Health and Social Security, Scottish Home and Health Department, and Welsh Office. (1969) Working Party on Management Structure in the Local Authority Nursing Services. *Report.* DHSS, London (Chairman E.L. Mayston).

Department of Health and Social Security (1972) *Management Arrangements for the Reorganised National Health Service.* HMSO, London (Chairman Sir P. Rogers).

Department of Health and Social Security and Welsh Office (1979) *Patients First: Consultative Paper on the Structure and Management of the National Health Service in England and Wales.* HMSO, London.

Department of Health and Social Security (1982) *NHS Reorganization: Unit Level Nursing Posts – Pay Grade Title.* DHSS, London (Advance letter (NM) 2/82).

Department of Health and Social Security (1982) *NHS Reorganization: Senior Nurse Posts.* DHSS, London (Advance letter (NM) 5/82).

Department of Health and Social Security (1982) *Nurses and Midwives Advisory Committee.* DHSS, London (DA (82) 2).

Glennerster, H., Owens, P. and Kimberley, A. (1986) *The Nursing Management Function after Griffiths in the North West Thames Region: an Interim Report.* London School of Economics and Political Science and North West Thames Regional Health Authority.

Hansard (1986a) National Health Service Management. *Hansard: House of Commons*, **93** (78), 14 Mar, 1318–30; **93** (78 pt2), 14 Mar, 1331–82.

Hansard (1986b) Nurses and the NHS reorganization. *Hansard: House of Lords*, **450** (108), 131–62.

Heyhoe, B. (1985) Letter to all regional health authority chairmen, 20 November.

Ministry of Health and Scottish Home and Health Department (1966) *Report of the Committee on Senior Nursing Staff Structure.* HMSO, London (Chairman B. Salmon).

NHS Managment Inquiry Team (1983) *NHS Management Inquiry: (letter to the secretary of state)* The Team, London (Team leader E.R. Griffiths).

Parliament (1979) *Nurses, Midwives and Health Visitors Act.* HMSO, London.

Secretary of State for Social Services (1972) *National Health Service Reorganisation: England.* HMSO, London.

United Kingdom Central Council for Nursing, Midwifery and Health Visiting (1984) *Code of Professional Conduct for the Nurse, Midwife and Health Visitor*, 2nd edn. UKCC, London.

United Kingdom Central Council for Nursing, Midwifery and Health Visiting (1986) *Project 2000: a New Preparation for Practice.* UKCC, London.

5 Nursing research: growth and development

CLAIRE GOODMAN

Research within nursing has developed over the last forty years from a minority activity to something which is recognized as essential for the growth and development of the profession. The research-aware nurse is one who can find and comprehend research literature and apply its findings to her area of practice. The research-based education curriculum is one that not only draws on available research as a basis for teaching but also encourages a questioning approach in the student.

THE GROWTH OF RESEARCH IN NURSING

In dwelling upon the vital importance of sound observation it must never be lost sight of what observation is for. It is not for the sake of miscellaneous information or curious facts, but for the sake of saving life and increasing health and comfort. (Nightingale, 1859)

It can be seen from this quote that Florence Nightingale was a firm believer in the value of applied research and that nurses could and should systematically collect information in order to plan and assess their care. As Seaman (1987) notes, in Nightingale's view devotion is useless without ready and correct observations. It is surprising therefore that this philosophy and approach to care did not generate within nursing an atmosphere conducive to research activity. It was not until after World War II that research within nursing first gained a foothold. There are many reasons why there should have been a dearth of nursing research in the post-Nightingale era. It could be argued that the structure and organization of nurse training plus the hierarchy of nursing itself, militated against a questioning approach to care and encouraged a reliance on rule keeping and known practice. Isabel Menzies (1960) in her classic work of the 1950s where she studied the nursing service within one general hospital, highlighted some of the characteristics of the nursing structure which in the past may have inhibited (and to an extent still do) the development of nursing research. She described the process of nursing which involved for example, ritual task-performance, avoidance of change and the idealization and under-estimation of personal developmental possibilities. Menzies (1960) argued that these were essentially defensive techniques which had developed over time in order to deal with the anxiety-provoking situations that nurses constantly encounter. She further observed that efforts to initiate serious change were often met with acute anxiety and hostility and that this resistance was directly attributable to the social defence mechanisms which had evolved over time. Whilst Menzies' work was not concerned with the development of research within nursing, it can be seen that the environment she described would not have been conducive to facilitating the research process which encourages a questioning approach and can stimulate change and challenge established practice. Nevertheless, it was in the 1940s and 1950s that changes within and without nursing combined to make it possible for nursing research to attract support, interest and official approval.

A series of commissioned reports in the 1940s to look into the needs of nursing education discussed the needs for nursing to have a more academic base. Both the Horder (RCN, 1943) and the Wood (Ministry of Health, 1947) reports explicitly and implicitly recommended the development of degree programmes in nursing. The idea for research into nursing was put forward by the Wood Report when it had found that few statistics were available for manpower planning and no formal evaluation of nurse education had been undertaken. The working party had been asked to examine the proper task of the nurse. As they had failed to resolve this issue they proposed a study should be undertaken on the work of the nurse. The Nuffield Provincial Hospitals Trust consequently undertook to make job analyses of the work of the hospital and public health nurses. As Rosemary White (1982) noted in her study of the period, 'Some of the profession after 1948 were caught up by the exciting prospect of research into their activities but other nurses thought that outside bodies might lack understanding of nursing values and pressures, these therefore wanted nurses to be involved'. This was an early indication that nurses were becoming aware of the potential importance and relevance of research for the profession.

Outwith nursing the growth of Social Science Departments in the universities and the increasing interest in the contribution of the behavioural sciences meant that researchers from outside were becoming interested in investigating the way health care provision was practised and managed. In the post-war years the changing status of women meant that they were more aware of the different educational opportunities open to them, especially university education. Many of the earliest nurse researchers were women who had trained as nurses and then undertaken either full-time or part-time higher education and had returned to nursing to apply the conceptual and theoretical frameworks of the social and behavioural sciences to issues of nursing management and practice.

For any type of research to be undertaken seriously it needs resources, both money and suitably qualified manpower to ensure its success. In 1952 Boots the Chemist funded a fellowship in nursing for seven years which was open to graduates and administered through the University of Edinburgh. Also in 1952, the Florence Nightingale Memorial Committee established the Dan Mason Research Trust. The purpose of this trust being to support research that investigated basic nursing education, methods of training and nursing techniques. These were some of the first sources of funding that were explicitly for the support of nurses undertaking research. In 1956 the Royal College of Nursing published a new policy on nursing: Observations and Objectives. This was designed to update the Horder Report and it confirmed not only the need for graduate nurses to take leadership posts but also for research into nursing. In that same year the College announced that Marjorie Simpson would undertake research into the development of nursing as a profession at the London School of Economics.

Bond and Bond (1982), see the development of the nursing departments within the universities as one of the key influences in the development of nursing research. The first academic department of nursing was established at Edinburgh University under the direction of Miss Elsie Stephenson and in 1960 four undergraduate students were admitted to the integrated degree course. This was soon followed by the setting up of a nursing department at Manchester University. Now there are approximately 15 universities and polytechnics offering nursing education to degree level as well as the opportunity to undertake full-time research with academic nursing supervision. Although some commentators had argued that the presence of academic departments of nursing only served to create an elite of nurse researchers whose goal is higher degrees and not necessarily (or primarily) the advancement of nursing, the influence of these departments has been significant in developing a more critical approach to nursing care and creating the expertise, and resources with which to describe, explain and when appropriate, change nursing.

Also in the 1960s a small group of nurses involved in nursing research on their own account, formed a self-help association. Different nursing specialties began to benefit from research that was specific to their needs and interests, for example, Lisbeth Hockey's (1966, 1968, 1972) series of surveys commissioned by the Queen's Institute of District Nursing into different aspects of the district nurse's role and work. Also Doreen Norton a ward sister at the time obtained funding into problems associated with the care of the elderly. As Rosemary White (1982) notes, Norton's work was one of the first pieces of research to demonstrate the merit of investigating nursing procedures as opposed to an earlier preoccupation with organization and manpower; a trend she claims which was not apparent until the late 1960s when the skills as opposed to the procedures needed for nursing became the focus for research.

In 1966 a working group of doctors, nurses, sociologists and civil servants were called together by the Department of Health and from this grouping emerged a research project: 'The Study of Nursing Care'. This was the first structured nursing research enterprise and proved to be a landmark in the development and establishment of nursing research. It was administered through the Royal College of Nursing and many seminal pieces of nursing research emerged from this particular project which ran until 1974.

In 1978/79 the Department of Health and Social Security awarded twelve fellowships with two being offered respectively by the Scottish and Northern Irish Department. These fellowships recognized the need for providing training in research methods and skills and enabled nurses interested in research to undertake studies with adequate academic supervision.

Simpson (1981), when reviewing the development of nursing research in Britain, indicated that whereas there had been a significant increase in the number of studies undertaken by nursing, in order to maintain continuous attention to particular aspects of nursing a coherent research programme is needed with sustained finance. She warns against the dangers of one-off studies which do not refer to previous studies or do not attempt to give a theoretical base to the work. The nursing research units which have been established go some way to initiate and sustain nursing research, the first having been established in 1971 in Edinburgh. Since then units based within the Universities of London, Surrey and Warwick have been established, concerned respectively with issues of nursing education, practice and policy.

Now, at the end of the 1980s, there is an increasing importance placed upon nursing research and it is not unreasonable to claim that it is an established feature of the profession. Increasingly, job descriptions are requiring that post holders not only keep up to date with recent research but also be willing to support and participate in research activity. Many district health authorities have nursing research posts and schools of nursing are increasingly recognizing the importance of threading research appreciation and understanding throughout the nursing curriculum. It can, therefore, be seen that the growth of nursing research in the post-war years has been meteoric, from the interest of the few to a priority for the policy makers within nursing. Although it is undeniable that much growth in a relatively short space of time is impressive, the question has to be asked to what extent has it influenced practice? Is the nursing profession only giving a grudging lip service to the need for a research base? What is the relationship between nursing research and practice, marriage or divorce?

THE RESEARCH AND PRACTICE DEBATE

Simpson (1981) argued that whilst it could be said that the development of nursing research could be said to have 'reached the end of the beginning, the relationship between research and practice remained elementary'. Earlier, Dickoff, James and Semradet (1975) referring to American nursing research, claimed that nursing practice was left largely untouched by research because researchers were so concerned with pseudotechnical research methodology that they lost sight of the real problems of nursing. In seeking to address this issue several authors both British and American have reviewed nursing research publications in an attempt to assess to what extent nursing research is concerned with issues specific to patient care.

O'Connel (1983) received a decade of American research papers that focused on the patient and included a nursing action as a variable. She found that only 28% (145), of the studies reviewed could be classified as research concerned with nursing practice. In these relatively little attention has been paid to physical needs despite the fact that the practice-based nurse spends much of her time meeting patient needs for cleanliness, medication, nutrition and pain relief. Fewer than 5% of the studies examined these topics with little detectable changes of emphasis over the ten years that were reviewed. Lelean (1981) reviewed 150 British studies mentioned in the DHSS nursing research abstracts and found that only 20% could be classified as dealing with practice issues. More recently, Wilson-Barnett (1986) examined ten years of research papers published in the *Journal of Advanced Nursing*. She found that from the beginning of the 1980s there was a definite rise in the number of studies directly relating to patient care. By way of explanation she suggested that in the past, nursing research tended to avoid practice issues partly because of their inherent complexity and partly because many of the earlier nurse researchers had a basis in sociology and social policy leading to a concern with administration and educational matters.

RESEARCH THAT IS READY FOR PRACTICE

So, is nursing research generating and validating the knowledge necessary for clinical nursing practice? Fawcett (1983) suggests several reasons as to why contemporary nursing research may not always be applicable or ready for the practice setting. Essentially, her arguments would seem to indicate that nursing research in many areas is not necessarily mature enough for implementation. For example, when examining the research approaches used by many nurse researchers they have been heavily influenced by the philosophy of other disciplines, particularly the social sciences. In other words there has been a tendency to use methods which have not been primarily developed to tackle nursing issues. Consequently, she argues it is not until the research approaches used become more specific to the science and needs of nursing that the greater the likelihood will be of its direct relevance for practice. Even taking this into consideration, Fawcett (1983) identifies a hierarchy of research development necessary for research findings to be able to transfer to the practice setting. Thus the first stage of research and the basis for the development of knowledge in any area of nursing interest is descriptive research which can classify and categorize phenomena. Then, once the essential characteristics of a study's variables have been identified research can begin to describe the relationships between key variables. It is only at this point that research findings can begin to have a relevance and application for nursing practice. From this one can develop research which through building on the preceding descriptive work can begin to focus on explanation and prediction, identifying goals for clinical practice which can be tested using experimental and practice-based research. It is, therefore, not so surprising given this schema of the development of research-based knowledge that it is only latterly that there has been an increase in the number of clinically based studies which are testing and evaluating different nursing approaches and innovations. By necessity, the earlier nursing research work was concerned with 'setting the scene' of nursing, describing what nurses do. These studies yielded a wealth of information about the activity of nursing, and they have provided the baseline information necessary for subsequent studies wishing to test particular nursing interventions. For the sake of the development of nursing knowledge which is relevant for practice it is important that nursing research does not become 'stuck' in only undertaking descriptive work, as there is an inherent danger when using only descriptive work that the deficiencies of nursing are highlighted without then going on to undertake research that seeks remedies or to improve care.

Another consideration when assessing how much of nursing research is ready for implementation into the practice setting is the extent to which the findings of one study can be said to be generalizable. It is only as work is replicated in different practice settings and with different populations that the nurse practitioner can be confident that the findings represent an integrated and thoroughly evaluated body of knowledge. The very fact that research findings often require change which in itself may necessitate an involvement of time, personnel expertise and equipment means that for the nurse it is only worthwhile going all out for change if he or she can be assured that it is going to produce meaningfully different results in patient care. Nursing only now is recognizing the need for building from descriptive stage research to that of evaluation. What is increasingly needed is a series of studies in specific areas which draw on the progress from previous work to establish a cohesive body of research evidence ready for transfer to the practice setting. There are areas of nursing where research has begun to influence thinking and practice. A few examples of where this has occurred include pressure area care, the development of the ward sister role and communication and information-giving skills. Pressure sore research has ranged from the classification of sores and assessment of their prevalence (Jordan and Barbenel, 1983), to the testing of preventive measures (Lowthian, 1982) and different treatment regimes.

The recognition of the importance of the ward sister has long-been acknowledged but seminal work by Pembrey (1980) began to identify the key functions of the role. A study by Lathlean and Farnish (1984) showed how the newly appointed sister could be trained and developed to maximize the role. Similarly, the now classic work of Hayward (1975), Boore (1978) and Wilson-Barnett (1978) pointed to the importance of information-giving as a factor in reducing anxiety and promoting recovery. More recent work focusing on nurses' communication skills (Clark, 1981; Faulkner, 1980) have demonstrated a need for skills training in this area and generated interest in the subject area as a whole amongst clinically involved nurses (Goodman, 1986). These diverse examples of nursing research indicate how research can gradually influence and be relevant for practice.

PROBLEMS OF IMPLEMENTATION

If it is accepted that nursing research has begun to reach a level of sophistication when it can be implemented and used for practice, to what extent have nurses been able to utilize research findings? It is a question which has exercised the minds of many nurses involved in research who are anxious that their findings should not be disregarded. Hunt (1981) in a much-quoted article discussed some of the reasons why findings that could have a direct leaning on nursing care are largely ignored. She suggests that one simple reason is that ward- and community-based nursing staff do not get to hear about relevant research because results are not disseminated. Frequent criticisms have been levelled at researchers who do not publicize their findings or make them readily available. Hopefully, this is becoming less of an issue although it is sometimes difficult to establish at what point the researcher's responsibilities to make known the findings ends, and the nurse's responsibility to keep abreast of relevant research begins. It is worth noting that Stapleton (1983), in seeking to identify the educational needs of ward sisters, also identified difficulty of access, for example to nursing libraries, as a barrier to using research findings. Hunt (1981), further suggested that nurses had difficulty understanding published studies. This points to a lack of preparation in research appreciation which until recently was a problem in nurse education. It is also not the nature of research to draw conclusions on findings without highlighting the limitations of a study or offering alternative interpretations to or caveats on results. Robinson (1987) suggests that researchers should be more directive as to how their research findings should be used and indicate what the implications are for their use in practice. The development of different research methods is important, as different approaches yield new insights and explanations of phenomena. There is a potential danger though, that the process and activity of research becomes of more interest than the results themselves, thereby risking alienating the very audience one most wants to reach. Furthermore, the language of research can be obscure with its own modes of expression and jargon. Researchers have a responsibility to ensure their work is readable without being patronizing.

A major influence on whether research findings are utilized or not, must be the incentive offered to nurses to make the effort to become research aware. The negative reasons for using research are obvious, that is the issue of the nurses' liability in engaging in practice that has no sound base, but what are the positive inducements? The profession may be giving only lip service support to the value of research in nursing if it is not actively creating opportunities for clinical nurses to become involved in further education and research nor offering positive recognition for nurses who are research literate and implementing findings. For example, how many health authorities make knowledge of relevant research a key criterion in the appointment of ward sisters or in the annual appraisal of nurse managers? It is not sufficient to make research mindedness a clause of a job description if no active support or recognition is offered. If research findings are to become a discussed and integral part of practice there needs to be more explicit support and structure within the health service. At present this occurs on an *ad hoc* basis for example with locally based research interest groups who meet to discuss current research. Weatherston (1981), in a discussion of how best to implement research, commented that it is a distinct possibility that the only way of creating meaningful liaison between practice and research is through nurses having active involvement in both areas so that the memories are fresh of the constraints and realities of service areas. As an example of how this may work White (1984) demonstrated the effectiveness of using research methods and findings to effect change in the clinical setting. Her study looked at the reasons for the high attrition rate in an obesity clinic. She found that whereas the staff emphasized fitness and wellness as positive outcomes of losing weight, the clients' primary reason for seeking to lose weight was to improve their body image. Health as an incentive was therefore a secondary issue. As a result of the study the clinic amended its approach and the attrition rate lowered. There is an increasing interest in the value of appointing clinical nurses who have an explicit research component to their job. It is an idea which has been more extensively developed in North America within the clinical nurse specialist role. These posts frequently require the nurse to be educated to Masters level. It is important when considering such appointments that sufficient time is given for research as it is a time-consuming activity which can easily be squeezed out with the other responsibilities and pressures of the combined role.

Overall, it can be seen that to develop in nurses the desire and skills to implement research findings there is a continuing but little-recognized need for support. The support comes through education, a receptive clinical environment that is amenable to change and through the creation of a career structure which formally recognizes the role of research and its relevance. Oberst (1985) in discussing the integration of research and clinical nursing roles made the following statement:

> For the clinician, this means learning to think about practice in new ways, a willingness to challenge old assumptions and to accept greater accountability, not just for one's personal practice but for the development of more broadly applicable knowledge as well. It will also require the development of new skills and the courage for the right to use them.

The researcher, too, will need to develop new ways of thinking about the practice/research interface. This means developing a tolerance for diversity of approaches creatively designing studies compatible with practice realities and learning to communicate in the language of practice as well as research.

FUTURE TRENDS: FUTURE NEEDS

Research: the quantitative, qualitative continuum

As nursing research has become established and more sophisticated there is an increasing interest in the variety of research approaches and their theoretical perspectives used to investigate nursing. Much of nursing research has used solely quantitative research methods, those which have a positivist approach. The quantitative 'scientific' method is derived largely from the natural sciences with the emphasis on controlling and manipulating data (Leininger, 1985). It is a deductive process of building up knowledge. As Duffy (1985) comments, the true experiment is the classic example of the quantitative, positivist approach. There is an assumption that the real world lends itself to objective measurement, that variables of human behaviour can be isolated, documented and qualified to allow statistical analysis and assessment of the probability of a particular outcome. From this process facts and causal relationships can be proposed. In an earlier part of this chapter when discussing the progressive and cumulative nature of research a positivist paradigm was assumed. More recently, the unassailable 'rightness' of this kind of research design has been challenged particularly when considering research which is seeking to explain not only what is occurring but also the meaning behind what is observed. Leininger (1985) is strongly opposed to quantitative research approaches which study people as reducible, measurable objects independent of historical, cultural and social contexts. She claims: 'Indeed, to reduce people and nursing practices to parts, machinelike operations or sensual empirical data, has never been cognisant with nursing's traditional values of personalised intimate, holistic and human services.' This kind of viewpoint has led to a developing discussion and interest in qualitative research approaches, as a means of explaining the complex phenomenon of nursing.

Leininger (1985) sees that the goal of qualitative research 'is to document and interpret as fully as possible the totality of whatever is being studied in particular contexts from the people's viewpoint or frame of references'. This includes the study, identification and analysis of subjective and objective data in order to understand the internal and external worlds of people. Disciplines which emphasize this type of research approach include anthropology, history, sociology and philosophy. Within British nursing research a number of studies have been undertaken using qualitative research designs in order to give meaning to what was being studied. For example, an early piece of research by Kratz (1978) used a modified form of an approach called grounded theory not only to describe district nurses' care of stroke patients in the community but also to interpret the meaning and value of that care to the district nurses. Melia (1981), sought to describe student nurses' experiences of nurse training. She achieved this through in-depth open interviews with student nurses. She did not bring to the interviews a set of preformed questions but allowed what the student nurses told her to direct the course of the interviews. From this emerged common experiences and conflicts which the students described and which Melia was able to categorize. She argued that this research approach was more valid as it enabled those being studied to describe the reality of nurse training as they saw it to 'tell it like it is'. They were not confined by the researcher's preconceived ideas. It is this valuing of the subjective which places this kind of research at the opposite end of the continuum from the experiment which strives for control, objectivity and tests of reliability. Greenwood (1984) challenged the value of some of the early nursing research which used experimental design in the ward setting. She argued that what was studied did not reflect the context and constraints of nursing because of the amount of researcher control and intervention needed to produce the results. She suggested this was a major reason for research findings not being seen as relevant or applicable for nurses, because the manner in which the research was conducted did not reflect reality. Greenwood (1984) went on to argue that action research was therefore the way forward for nursing research. Action research is an approach which can employ many different research techniques, for example, observation, interviews, retrospective analysis of documents. It is an evaluating research approach which involves those being studied from the start when research problems are being identified throughout the period of the intervention right up to the final conclusions. The researcher works in collaboration and co-operation with those being studied. Lathlean and Farnish (1984) used an action research approach to evaluate the introduction of a ward sister training programme, and showed how it was possible to adapt and respond to situations that arose during the study as part of the action research process.

In much of the debate about qualitative and quantitative research it can be misleading to talk as though faced with an either/or option. Qualitative research approaches can be more appropriately applied to certain types of research problems than to others, and in many situations in conjunction with quantitative research approaches. Polit and Hungler (1983), suggest some major purposes for qualitative techniques to describe when little is known about a phenomenon, group or institution; to generate a hypothesis where observation generates ideas which can then be tested and re-examined; and when seeking to understand relationships and causal processes. For whilst quantitative methods may demonstrate that variables are systematically related to one another, alone they may fail to provide insights as to why the variables are related. Finally, qualitative material can be useful to illustrate the findings of a quantitatively focused study. As Leininger (1985) has commented, qualitative research findings can be of considerable benefit to quantitative studies in that the findings 'put the flesh on' and give meaning to statistical or numerical findings.

That nursing research is able to adopt methods on the basis of their appropriateness for a given situation and is not constrained by a rigid adherence to one research approach is indicative of an increasing professional self-confidence. Qualitative research requires a high level of sophistication and analytical expertise in the researcher and the importance placed on subjectivity does not infer a lack of vigour. Quantitative and qualitative research approaches lie along a continuum and do not occupy opposing camps. As research in nursing continues to develop a methodology that is responsive to the complexity of nursing care, so a database will grow which is distinctively nursing knowledge.

The funding market for nursing research

Earlier in the chapter when discussing the growth of research in nursing it was apparent that nursing research began to take hold once money became available not only to fund full-time researchers but also projects that were of several years' duration. The financing of research is central to its advancement; without time and resources research activity dies. There are several sources, actually and theoretically, available to nurses for financial support. Central government funding has proved to be the main support of nursing research. It currently funds two of the three research units in England, and the Scottish Home and Health Department support an equivalent nursing research unit in Edinburgh. Over the years the DHSS has made available nursing research studentships to enable nurses to undertake full-time research for a higher degree and simultaneously receive some research training. In addition to this individual projects of particular interest to current national policy or debate have been funded often for two to three years. Salter (1985) in reviewing government funding of nursing research warns that nursing has placed too much reliance on this one source of support. Furthermore, whilst this support has been fairly constant over the years as a percentage of total government research funding nursing projects account for very little. In the recent past the availability of funds specifically for nursing research has been contracting. Currently, for England and Wales there are only three full-time nursing research studentships available, where in previous years there have been more than ten offered at a given time.

The Locally Organized Research Scheme is a source of funding administered through regional health authorities and designed to encourage research among health service employees, particularly those relatively new to the activity. This is a major source of funding which is theoretically readily available for nurses. Nationally, however, there is little uptake by nurses. Few proposals are submitted and those that are, are often not of sufficient calibre to attract support. In all the regions medical research receives the bulk of the funding although many of the committees have specifically expressed a desire to support nursing research. There are two issues which nursing has to address in relation to this particular scheme. First, to ensure that nurses working within the NHS are aware of the scheme as a potential funding source for nursing and not solely medicine. Second, to obtain advice and training in the submission of research proposals, a particular skill which takes more time than can often be allowed within a full-time clinical job.

Charitable foundations have funded nursing research in the past, although there is not a picture of consistent or sustained support. However, some of the cancer charities are now recognizing the importance of research into the education and practice of nursing cancer patients. The King Edward's Hospital Fund has joint-funded several key nursing projects. It would seem that many charities are open to nursing research applications but do not have a tradition of providing support. Similarly, nurses may have been hesitant in pursuing this as a possible avenue of funding. Salter (1985) points out that as there is an increasing interest in obtaining value for money, nursing potentially has much to offer. The sheer size of the workforce demonstrates the impact a piece of nursing research into an aspect of patient care could have if findings were widely and efficiently disseminated. It is a proposition which is likely to be attractive to funding agencies and one that nurses should be ready to exploit.

Other possible sources of funding include the Health Education Authority, the Medical Research Council (MRC) and industry. It is noticeable that research and development for nursing is seldom seen as a necessary component of budgeting a health service within a district health authority. And yet, where nursing research posts have been created and money made available for district based research, nursing-led innovations have been possible. This may lead to economy but, more importantly, acknowledges the importance of nursing care and improved job satisfaction. Since the management reorganization of the National Health Service (Griffiths Report, NHS 1983) there is an explicit interest in standards of care. There is an opportunity for nursing to demonstrate how research into aspects of patient care can have implications for setting standards.

Obtaining financial support for research can be an uphill struggle, particularly as, apart from central government sources, there is not a strong tradition of nursing research support. Nevertheless, there are sources as yet relatively untapped which nurse researchers need to explore further and exploit.

FUTURE ISSUES

The barriers to nurses using research findings have already briefly been discussed, and they centre around relevance, accessibility and providing an environment which fosters research interest.

Now that research as an activity is more established, researchers should be wary of undertaking research which can only offer negative findings and highlight nurses' shortcomings. It is understandably disheartening to read about where we have an inadequate knowledge base or area of practice if no positive alternatives are offered. For example, one study by Seers (1987) highlighted that a significant number of postoperative patients were experiencing more pain than the nurses realized. In a video made to publicize these findings (Seers and Goodman, 1987), the accompanying booklet stressed that the aim was not to demonstrate how bad nurses were but to show the tremendous potential for effective pain management, and the insight the research could give nurses on patients' experiences. Nevertheless, there is a great need for further research in this area to further help nurses develop strategies of pain management that have a rational basis.

There is a danger that nursing research will become too introspective. Much of nursing activity is complementary to and interdependent with medicine. The development of multidisciplinary research needs more attention. Understandably, in the past nurse researchers have fought shy of too-close collaboration for fear of medical domination with nurses undertaking only the data collection component of the research. There is a clear need for more research-based dialogue between doctors and nurses and the commissioning of jointly led research projects. Many doctors do not appreciate being told that they work to a medical model which focuses only on the disease whereas nursing research has an holistic approach to the patient. The shared goal for medical and nursing research is, or should be, improved patient care therefore there is a greater likelihood for implementation of findings if there is collaboration.

Future proposed changes in the educational structure of nursing, if they occur, are likely to encourage research development. The only concern is that the subject matter of the research moves away from the clinical setting. With the current emphasis though on the need for a clinical career grading structure, and the interest in such innovations as the nursing development unit described by Pearson (1983), this is possibly not a serious worry.

CONCLUSION

In this chapter a brief overview has been attempted of the growth and development of nursing research and some of the issues that currently concern it. It is encouraging to see the diversity of research activity undertaken in the United Kingdom and the increasing importance placed upon it within education and to a lesser extent practice.

To attempt to chart nursing research as a topic alone within one chapter inevitably means that many issues are left untouched. Perhaps the days are numbered when one can talk about nursing research as a single entity or subject. It represents such a variety of interest and approaches.

Nursing should take encouragement from what has been achieved in a relatively short space of time. The responsibility now for the researcher, educator and practitioner alike is to ensure that findings are known, understood, implemented and further research questions asked which are grounded in the needs of the practice setting.

REFERENCES

Bond, S. and Bond, J. (1982) *Clinical Nursing Research Priorities: a Delphi Survey.* Health Care Research Unit, University of Newcastle on Tyne and Northern Regional Health Authority, Newcastle on Tyne.

Boore, J. (1978) *Prescription for Recovery.* Royal College of Nursing, London.

Clark, J.M. (1981) Communication in nursing. *Nursing Times,* **77**, 1 Jan 12–18.

Dickoff, J., James, P. and Semradet, J. (1975) Research: a stance for nursing research – tenacity or inquiry? Part 1. *Nursing Research,* **24**(2) Mar/Apr 84–8.

Duffy, M.E. (1985) Designing nursing research: the qualitative–quantitative debate. *Journal of Advanced Nursing,* **10**(3) May 225–32.

Faulkner, A. (1980) Communication and the nurse. *Nursing Times,* **76**, 4 Sep, Occasional Papers, 93–5.

Fawcett, J. (1983) Contemporary nursing research: its relevance to nursing practice, in *The Nursing Profession: A Time to Speak* (ed. N. Chaska, McGraw-Hill, New York.

Goodman, C. (1986) *A Delphi Survey of Clinical Nursing Research Priorities within a Regional Health Authority.* Unpublished MSc thesis, University of London.

Greenwood, J. (1984) Nursing research: a position paper. *Journal of Advanced Nursing,* **9**(1) Jan, 77–82.

Hayward, J. (1975) *Information – a Prescription against Pain.* Royal College of Nursing, London.

Hockey, L. (1966) *Feeling the Pulse.* Queen's Institute of District Nursing, London.

Hockey, L. (1968) *Care in the Balance.* Queen's Institute of District Nursing, London.

Hockey, L. (1972) *Use or Abuse?* Queen's Institute of District Nursing, London.

Hunt, J. (1981) Indicators for nursing practice: the use of research findings, *Journal of Advanced Nursing,* **6**(3) May, 189–94.

Jordan, M.M. and Barbenel, J.C. (1983) Pressure sore prevalence, in *Pressure Sores* (eds J.C. Barbenel, C.D. Forbes and G.D.O. Lowe) Macmillan, London.

Kratz, C.R. (1978) *Care of the Long Term Sick in the Community.* Churchill Livingstone, Edinburgh.

Lathlean, J. and Farnish, S. (1984) *The Ward Sister Training Project.* Nursing Education Research Unit, University of London, London (NERU report no. 3).

Leininger, M. (ed.) (1985) *Qualitative Research Methods in Nursing.* Grune and Stratton, Orlando, FL.

Lelean, S.R. (1981) Nursing research and higher education. *Journal of Advanced Nursing,* **6**(3) May, 240–1.

Lowthian, P. (1982) A review of pressure sore pathogenesis. *Nursing*

Times, **78**, 20 Jan, 117–21.

Melia, K. (1981) Communication in nursing 3. Student nurses' construction of nursing: a discussion of a qualitative method. *Nursing Times*, **77**, 16 Apr, 697–9.

Menzies, I.E.P. (1960) A case study in the functioning of social systems as a defence against anxiety. *Human Relations*, **13**, 95–121.

Ministry of Health, Department of Health for Scotland and Ministry of Labour and National Service (1947) *Report of the working party on the recruitment and training of nurses.* HMSO, London (Chairman Sir Robert Wood).

NHS Management Inquiry Team (1983) NHS management inquiry: (letter to the Secretary of State) The Team, London (Team leader E.R. Griffiths).

Nightingale, F. (1859) *Notes on Nursing.* Harrison, London.

Oberst, M.T. (1985) Integrating research and clinical practice roles. *Topics in Clinical Nursing*, **7**(2) Jul, 45–53.

O'Connel, K. (1983) Nursing practice: a decade of research, in *The Nursing Profession: a Time to Speak* (ed. N. Chaska), McGraw-Hill, New York.

Pearson, A. (1983) *The Clinical Nursing Unit.* Heinemann Medical, London.

Pembrey, S. (1980) *The Ward Sister – Key to Nursing.* Royal College of Nursing, London.

Polit, D. and Hungler, B. (1983) *Nursing Research: Principles and Methods*, 2nd edn, Lippincott, Philadelphia, PA.

Robinson, J. (1987) The relevance of research to the ward sister. *Journal of Advanced Nursing*, **12**(4) Jul, 421–9.

Royal College of Nursing, Nursing Reconstruction Committee (1943) *Report. Section 2, education and training, Section 3, recruitment.* Royal College of Nursing, London (Chairman Lord Horder).

Salter, B. (1985) The funding market for nursing research. *Journal of Advanced Nursing*, **10**(2) Mar, 155–63.

Seaman, C. (1987) *Research Methods: Principles, Practice and Theory for Nursing*, 3rd edn, Appleton and Lange, Norwalk, Conn.

Seers, C.J. (1987) *Pain anxiety and recovery in patients undergoing surgery.* Unpublished PhD thesis, King's College, University of London.

Seers, C.J. and Goodman, C. (1987) Perceptions of pain. *Nursing Times*, **83**, 2 Dec, 37–8.

Simpson, M. (1981) Current issues in nursing research, in *Current Issues in Nursing* (ed. L. Hockey), Churchill Livingstone, Edinburgh.

Stapleton, M. (1983) *Ward Sisters – Another Perspective.* Royal College of Nursing, London.

Weatherston, L. (1981) Bridging the gap: liaison between nursing education and nursing service. *Journal of Advanced Nursing*, **6**(2) Mar, 147–52.

White, J.H. (1984) The relationship of clinical practice and research. *Journal of Advanced Nursing*, **9**(2) Mar, 181–7.

White, R. (1982) *The effects of the NHS on the nursing profession.* Unpublished PhD thesis, University of Manchester.

Wilson-Barnett, J. (1978) Patients' emotional response to barium x-rays. *Journal of Advanced Nursing,* **3**(1) Jan/Feb, 37–46.

Wilson-Barnett, J. (1981) Assessment of recovery with special reference to a study with post-operative cardiac patients. *Journal of Advanced Nursing,* **6**(6) Nov, 435–45.

Wilson-Barnett, J. (1986) *Research: its Relationship to Practice and Representation in the Journal of Advanced Nursing.* North West Thames Nursing Research Conference, King's College, University of London.

6 Nursing and politics: the unquiet relationship

TREVOR CLAY

There are still a few nursing leaders for whom participation in the political process is totally alien. For them the words nursing, power and politics are incompatible. They have transmitted these values to thousands of nurses under their direction. This is a frightening situation in the United Kingdom where, more than any other country in the world, politicians have a direct impact on the entire health and nursing service.

Since the establishment of the National Health Service (NHS) in July 1948 the scale, direction and development of nursing has been firmly under the guidance of the politicians. Reforms or new initiatives in pay and conditions, education or even the nursing hierarchy have all been dependent on political debate and consent before change has been initiated. The failure to acknowledge this has been one of the main obstacles to progress in nursing for over three decades.

Yet the majority of nurses in the United Kingdom successfully convinced themselves that their future lay outside politics, that they could stand aside from the arguments in government, parliament and the press which decided the future for nursing. It was a truly remarkable situation which for almost thirty years gave credence to the arguments that nursing should not become politically involved.

Nurses pay in 1987/88 amounted to £4300 million from a public expenditure budget of £154 billion. When other nursing costs such as education are added to the bill, it amounts to almost 3% of public expenditure in the UK (Review Body for Nursing Staff, Midwives, Health Visitors and Professions Allied to Nursing, 1987). It is an illusion that any Prime Minister or politician is going to be indifferent to the spending of such vast sums of money amounting to £3 out of every £100 collected in taxation. In the health departments it amounts to almost 30% of total expenditure and for the Secretary of State at the Department of Health and Social Security (DHSS) it amounts to almost 20% of his total health and personal social services budget. While the sums have changed since 1948 the realities for the politicians have not. What happened to nursing affected their whole ability to control health expenditure and direction and could not be ignored.

Yet the illusion persisted. This was only possible because of the particular circumstances which existed from 1948 until the late 1970s. During the whole of that time there was a clear political consensus among the parties in government that the NHS was a good and worthwhile thing to be invested in for the benefit of the whole society. From 1948 until the end of the Callaghan government in 1979 the NHS consistently experienced growth and investment by governments of both parties which exceeded the growth in the economy. This experience of growth within a political consensus insulated nursing and its leaders. It felt as though there was no political interference, no control. The control, however, was there but the consensus made it appear benevolent. The strings were there but they were not obvious.

The consensus on the worth of the NHS also produced the tendency for government to concede to the health professionals a considerable degree of autonomy in the running and development of the service. The epitome of this was reached after the 1974 reorganization when consensus management was established with health authorities effectively being run by agreement among the doctors, nurses, administrators and treasurers. Before any major change was made the health professionals, including nurses, could expect to be consulted and could largely expect their views to be heeded. For the nursing leaders at national level this relationship appeared to be a direct one with the government health departments which did not require the involvement of parliament or engagement with politicians or political parties.

The debate between the health service and the government was itself dominated by debate between the medical profession and politicians and was generally about administrative reorganization rather than clinical issues affecting the delivery of care. The issues which hit the headlines were from the agenda set by medicine. Nursing was seen, and often saw itself, as somewhat secondary in the debate.

While the NHS was a radical and exciting step the price of that radical change was the wholesale transfer of the traditions, culture and hierarchy of the old hospital system into the new NHS and in that change the nursing hierarchy was secondary.

There was a model of political involvement for nurses but it was one which not many found attractive. This was the trade union movement. This model tended to copy the activities of the industrial trade unions, using strike action and confrontation techniques very alien to a caring service; alien also to a service built on religious and military structures and values. The trade unions, the National Union of Public Employees (NUPE) and the Confederation of Health Service Employees (COHSE), were affiliated to one political party, the Labour Party. Until the massive expansion of the Royal College of Nursing in the late 1970s and 1980s the majority of the nursing workforce remained non-unionized. COHSE has always had a strong base in the old institutions for mental illness and mental handicap, but recruitment outside those traditional areas had always been weak. The Royal College of Nursing (RCN) which in 1987 was the ninth largest trade union in the United Kingdom and organized 70% of qualified nurses, was in the 1950s and 1960s a much smaller organization dominated by the views and leadership of traditional managers and educators. The consequence of all this was that nursing leaders remained largely out of contact with any of the major political networks which have so influenced other 'professional' groupings in society such as teachers and civil servants.

The 1970s saw a series of events which shook the insularity which had kept nurses out of the political process and forced a re-examination of the position.

Although there had been problems in the previous decades over attempts to reform nursing education both in 1947 (Wood, Ministry of Health, 1947) and 1964 (Platt, RCN, 1964) and with pay and management in the 1960s, none had been severe enough to provoke the re-assessment which was to take place in the 1970s.

The first significant crisis was over pay when in 1974 the RCN went so far as to threaten mass resignations from nurses unless the problems of nurses' pay were tackled. The Secretary of State of the day, Barbara Castle, established an inquiry under Lord Halsbury which duly reported and awarded significant increases in pay. These gains, however, were quickly eroded in the high inflation of the mid-1970s and by various forms of pay restraint and control.

The financial crisis of 1976, with the severe restrictions on capital expenditure imposed by the Chancellor, Dennis Healey, indicated decisively that the NHS would no longer be insulated from general economic considerations and therefore would not continue with unlimited growth led by demand.

In 1975 Mrs Thatcher was elected as leader of the Conservative Party. So began a process which would end the consensus between the political parties, not just on the NHS but on the whole role of the welfare state in society. The reassessment had been accelerated with attempts by Barbara Castle as Secretary of State to end all private medicine and private beds within the framework of the NHS. The debate about freedom of choice which this move provoked was to represent a sea change in attitudes towards the NHS among whole sections of conservative political opinion in the UK.

The debate about health-care provision itself was changing in the UK as it was in other countries. When the NHS had been established in 1948 the politicians had genuinely believed that, following a brief period of expansion to deal with immediate sickness, the costs of health care would go down as the general health of the population improved. This has clearly not been the case. Advances in medicine and the rising cost of medical technology raced ahead of all predictions. The nation's health did improve enormously with the virtual eradication of childhood diseases and scourges such as polio and tuberculosis.

The most expensive human condition for the health service is old age. Success in eradicating those diseases which had terminated life early merely helped people reach the age when more chronic and expensive diseases manifested themselves. The average cost to the NHS of a 30-year-old man in the UK in 1987 was around £180 per year. The average cost of a man over 75 years of age was

£1420 per year (Treasury, 1987). All the demographic trends up to the year 2000 show a dramatic increase in the numbers of elderly people. Economists and politicians faced with huge public expenditure deficits began to wonder aloud if the public purse could afford the expense.

The 1970s saw the rise of consumerism in health care as in other areas. The Patients Associations became more vocal; the public began to question the medical profession. A series of drug scandals, in particular with thalidomide, undermined public confidence. Decisions which had been left to the professions were debated in public and the assumption that the professional opinion was always right was seriously challenged.

Added to this financial, political, economic and social upheaval was a significant change in nurses themselves. The events of 1974 started a process which was to accelerate for the rest of the decade. The unionization of nurses was underway. The old divisions between the RCN and NUPE and COHSE were being eroded by the changing character of the RCN membership. Government trade union legislation in 1975 had forced the RCN to face up to trade union status or risk losing the privileges the legislation conferred upon certificated trade unions. In 1977 the RCN finally became certificated.

Behind this change was a growing confidence and assertiveness among women in society; an organization with over 90% of its members women could not be immune. The rate of growth in the RCN's membership indicated that trade unionism did have something to offer these individuals, but that they preferred the guarantee that it would not resort to the industrial model of trade unionism and the withdrawal of labour.

The events of the 'Winter of discontent' in 1978/79 signalled the start of a search for an alternative form of protest activity. The RCN even went so far as to establish a committee of its council under the chairmanship of June Clark to look at alternatives to industrial action which might constitute 'professional action'. Despite looking at all the permutations, it did not come up with proposals that could be effective in the narrow arena of employer and employee relations without affecting the quality of service to patients and breaking the pact which nurses have with society.

The winter of discontent produced the Clegg Commission Report (1980) and the pay awards of 1980 which included the reduction of the working week to 37.5 hours. But the gains were to be short-lived as inflation soared once again. In the winter of discontent the nurses, especially those in the RCN, had looked over the edge at industrial action and concluded that it was not an option. In 1980 it was still not clear what the best road would be.

The year 1979 saw change of another sort for the profession. The passing of the 1979 Nurses, Midwives and Health Visitors Act (Parliament, 1979) established the United Kingdom Central Council for Nursing, Midwifery and Health Visiting (UKCC) to replace the nine previous statutory and educational bodies. The process around the passing of this legislation revealed another side to politics in nursing: the potential for self-destruction which existed in the profession.

The changes in the nursing statutory bodies had been recommended as part of the Briggs Report in 1972 (Committee on Nursing, 1972). The Labour Government had brought forward legislation to enact the establishment of the new UKCC but so intense were the sectional interests inside nursing that the bill was only just passed at the eleventh hour before the 1979 election. Sectional interests are enshrined in the title and were reflected even more deeply in the membership of the council and the boards.

While nursing did not consciously enter the political arena systematically to engage politicians for reform until recently, there was a long tradition of sectional interests speaking out publicly to destroy the prospects of change. The prerequisite for effective political participation by a profession is the ability to speak with one voice in public. The medical profession is testimony to that reality. It is a lesson the branches of nursing have yet to learn and one of the main reasons for political ineffectiveness.

There are issues which society cannot leave to a single profession alone. The reform of nursing education is one of them. The general behaviour of branches of nursing over the reform of nursing education suggests that even in 1989 there is not a widespread realization that the rest of society has a say in the future of the thousands of young women and men who enter nursing every year and that reform in nursing education cannot ignore changes in society and educational thinking.

Any profession which takes over 26 000 young people each year, accounting for almost one-quarter of the qualified young women with between 5 'O' and 2 'A' levels, must have regard for the general, social and political debates about educational opportunities. These must be balanced between the narrow needs of the service and the rights of the individual to fair treatment and a decent education. When the UKCC published its proposals for the reform of nursing education in May 1986, many behaved as though the argument would be won or lost inside nursing. They seemed unaware that there were policy makers and many other NHS interested parties watching and waiting to exploit any divisions, as well as wanting to put forward their views.

For over 40 years it has been recognized that the existing model of nurse training was increasingly inappropriate. In 1986 6000 young people a year dropped out of training: such numbers demonstrate what had become a national scandal. The complex development of health care has made the presence of the student nurse as a worker on the wards increasingly stressful, as well as dangerous for the patients. With student nurses giving 60% of their time to work rather than education or training, it is not even a model which would have been approved by the majority of industrial training boards as satisfactory and would be regarded by most educationalists as prehistoric. Yet political isolation has characterized much of the debate as it has done in the past with exaggerated claims that reform of nurse education would make the student too academic or that he/she would have learned from books but totally lacked experience.

In February 1987 when the UKCC put its proposals to government, many expected that to be the end of the debate. In truth it was only the beginning. On 6 March 1987 Health Ministers sent the proposals to Health Authorities and Boards and the medical profession for consultation. By March 1988 the government had still not made up its mind about the proposals. Its major concern was the cost implications and the manpower problems the NHS faced, but also the extreme conservatism of the NHS on issues affecting change in the organization of nursing.

The debate on Project 2000 has been preceded by four major reports since the Second World War. The Wood report in 1947 recommended that students should be separated from employee status while they received their nursing education. The arguments for and against this proposal bear a striking similarity to those advanced today. A nursing shortage led to fears that student labour on the wards would be irreplaceable. Sectional interests were fighting for control over student nurses and unwilling to give up direct control or release them from the service. The 1949 Nurses Act was supposed to put some of the ideas of Wood into practice, but in reality few of the proposals were actually achieved. The matrons with their full managerial control of the nursing workforce combined, both inside the RCN and in the General Nursing Councils, to stifle proposals which lessened their control over student nurses.

The RCN turned to the subject again in 1961 when it established an inquiry into nursing education under the chairmanship of Sir Harry Platt. Again the proposal for supernumerary status was advanced and again the proposal was lost almost as soon as it emerged from the corridors of nursing into the political light. Instead, a separate report, which was meant to be taken side by side with Platt, 'Administering the Hospital Nursing Service – A Review', went forward politically and culminated in the Salmon Report of 1966 (Ministry of Health, 1966).

With both Wood and Platt nursing had been unable to envisage a process of political change. As soon as the proposals were announced they were destroyed by nursing itself with plenty of encouragement from traditional forces in medicine and administration opposed to nursing reform.

The reform of the administration and management of nursing went forward via the Salmon report. That reform had supporters in the general political arena. It was comprehensible to administrators, public and politicians alike and followed society's usual behaviour of seeking structural change to cure all ills.

As though nursing had learned nothing from its past, the same cycle occurred with the Briggs Committee Report on Nursing in 1972. It recommended major reforms in nursing education. Its recommendations for changes in the statutory framework have gone forward, though not as originally proposed, and only after the most extensive public display of sectional interest in the passing of the legislation in 1979. History was repeating itself for the third time.

Exasperated with the slow progress of proposals for the reform of nursing education, the RCN Council set up its own Commission on Nursing Education in December 1983 which reported in May 1985 under the chairmanship of Dr Harry Judge, Director of the Department of Educational Studies at the University of Oxford.

Again the proposal was advanced that nursing education should be separated from service provision and that student nurses should be supernumerary. At the time of the Judge Report in 1985 nursing was virtually the last major profession and certainly the largest, which had failed to share in the educational reforms of the 1960s and 1970s. Virtually all the professions allied to medicine had moved into further and higher education for their preparation. The nursing profession likes to reassure itself that this is because of the size and cost of nursing and that politicians will always put the most important issues off until last, because these tend to be the most difficult. While there is some truth in the claim that the scale of change involved in nurse education makes politicians more nervous than usual, the general thesis cannot stand examination. In 40 years nursing has had four major reports prior to Project 2000 and on each occasion has been over-cautious and sectional in its attitude. Politicians have merely exploited that fact. It will be a test of political maturity in nursing to see if Project 2000 can avoid the same fate, secure the necessary resources and be implemented according to the timetable set out by the UKCC.

While nursing has constructed a labyrinth of internal politics, it has proved consistently inept when it has ventured into the area of governmental politics. This is not to say that all nursing leaders are or have been inept. If that was the case, then the various reports would never have been commissioned at all. But the weight of conservative and sectional interests has consistently held back the most valiant efforts by previous leaders to initiate change.

In 1988 nursing faces a challenge about its future which cannot be avoided. The nursing shortage is qualitatively different in 1988 from any previous period. The NHS is not in a period of growth which can compensate for problems and create a sense of progress while aspects like nurse education stand still. In the shortages of the 1950s the NHS was able to resort to immigration for recruits, particularly in the West Indies. When the expansion of the hospitals in the late 1960s and early 1970s demanded more nursing manpower, it coincided with the products of the post-war baby boom. As that population bulge began to tail off in the late 1970s and early 1980s the bleak employment prospects for young people ensured that nursing, with an open door, enjoyed the pick of the crop. That is now changing dramatically and nursing is failing to get the recruits to fill places for which it had multiple applications only three or four years previously.

The system of nursing in the UK is based on high recruitment, low salaries and high turnover. The system works so long as recruits keep arriving at the door in enough numbers. This is the only way a system which loses 30000 whole-time equivalents and 6000 student nurses per year can survive. The system is clearly failing to achieve this while also failing to retain staff.

The unquiet relationship between nursing and the government may be about to change in a way few realise. Brought up in a generation used to pressing ideas on a reluctant government, few are ready for the notion that government itself may propose changes to nursing, independent of ideas generated inside the profession. Such an intervention may be government's response to the developing crisis in the nursing service in the NHS. Already it is pressing the case for more support workers and the extension of the Youth Training Schemes in clinical areas. The implications of this are a dilution of the ratio of trained to untrained staff. The enrolled nurse grade may be continued into the 1990s despite the inappropriateness of the training for the health needs of the next century. And student nurses may continue to be used as 'pairs of hands' on the wards. Whatever the outcome, no-one in 1988 can be in any doubt that the final decisions will not be taken solely by the profession itself but by politicians weighing up the many external factors which make up the full political climate in which the NHS now operates.

The greatest engine for change in the relationship between nursing and politics has been the issue of nurses' pay. The pay problems of the late 1960s, and in particular the problems which led to the establishment of Halsbury in 1974 (DHSS, 1974), were the most visible points where nursing issues became intensely political. It is said that Harold Macmillan advised his cabinet that there were three sets of people a politician should never fall out with: the miners, the Catholic Church and the nurses. It has yet to be seen whether Mrs Thatcher's government will keep to that dictum.

The winter of discontent in 1978 has led nurses to examine permutations on the industrial model of activity designed to force change from the employers: the government. Nurses had rejected that path. Trouble was to flare again in 1982 as the value of nurses' pay after Clegg in 1980 was quickly eroded by inflation. As with the reform of nursing education, changes in the statutory and administrative arrangements for nurses' pay had gone through a series of cycles repeating the same mistakes on each occasion. In 1968 the Whitley system of negotiation proved inadequate and the issue had to be referred to the then National Board for Prices and Incomes. Its recommended increase was a catching-up exercise soon undermined by inflation and overtaken by other groups. In 1974 Whitley broke down again and an inquiry was established under Lord Halsbury. Again the advances were quickly eroded. The winter of discontent in 1978/9 produced another breakdown in the Whitley system and the matter was passed to the Clegg Commission which gave nurses a shorter working week and a boost in pay. The inflation of 1981/2 again brought breakdown in 1982 and a long and protracted dispute in the NHS lasting eight months.

On two occasions during the 1982 dispute the government made a differential offer to nurses which was ahead of that being offered to other NHS workers. On both occasions in July and August (after ballots in the RCN and other organizations) nurses refused to accept the offer. Finally nurses began to see that it was necessary to break out of the repetitive cycle. Each year there was a major public interest at stake and a mechanism was needed to ensure progress from year to year rather than the rushed catching-up exercises of previous rounds.

In 1982 the realization dawned upon many in nursing that what had moved government to settle the nurses' pay issues, and what has pressurized them since in a way that no industrial action has succeeded in doing, is the public pressure, the democratic pressure that a major group of public sector workers can bring on government. In 1982 the industrial action produced a stalemate and a great deal of diversionary headlines about the issues of nurses striking rather than the merits of their case. What moved the issue forward was the effect of the nurses' pay ballots and the growing public support which the nursing stand commanded.

It is this experience which was to lead the then President of the RCN, Dame Sheila Quinn, to urge nurses to 'get political but stay professional' (1985). The unquiet relationship has changed again. As nursing found more and more doors closed at national level and, like all professional groups, found that there was nothing guaranteed about its views being heeded, it recognized the need for wider debate involving politicians. The need to make alliances with outside groups increased. The need for greater self discipline among nurses became apparent.

At the beginning of 1989 it is clear that political participation by nurses is to be tested to the full in the near future. The way in which the unquiet relationship has changed will be judged by the outcome of a series of debates which are about to take place. It is a long list and the fact that all these nursing issues are at the top of the political agenda is a testimony to the changes which have already taken place in nursing since 1982.

Project 2000 has reached the point where ministers and civil servants have to make choices. To have reached this point is an achievement in itself, unmatched in 40 years in the NHS.

In primary health care the government is confronted with amendments to the Health and Medicines Bill which propose the introduction of nurses prescribing and the nurse practitioner in the UK and a debate generated by the Cumberlege Report on Community Nursing (DHSS, 1986) which puts nurses to the forefront of a debate which politicians and doctors assumed would be confined to the old lines of general medical practice. Many are clearly still shocked at the force of the nursing intervention and its claim to an independent frontline role in the delivery of primary health care.

The government has been forced into a position where it acknowledges the character of the nursing shortage in terms dictated by the nursing profession. It has had to concede a clinical grading system which acknowledges more nursing dimensions than the crude system of pay flexibility being argued for by most NHS managers.

On basic nurses' pay the government is unable to counter the evidence about nursing shortages and is committed to the Review Body system. This has consistently delivered recommendations better than could have been negotiated, even in the pre-election year of 1987, in traditional pay bargaining with a government department.

But this move towards active political participation faces two major challenges in 1988. The first comes in the form of renewed industrial action, born out of frustration, by some nurses in NUPE and COHSE. The second is that the debate on the NHS and the headlines over nurses taking industrial action have provided a platform for those who wish to review the fundamental principles of the NHS to demand change and radical reform.

If nurses ever doubted the importance of political activity and participation, there can be no clearer case than when industrial action is presented as being the only course of effective action. Nurses are now faced with a review of the NHS which threatens its continuation as a national service, funded from taxation, comprehensive and free at the point of need. If this combination of events does not bring nurses out of their shell politically, then nothing will.

The relationship between government and the nursing profession is going through swift change. On the nursing side there is a growing recognition that public sector professional and trade union organizations cannot mimic the industrial model of trade unionism. In the unquiet relationship with government there is not a profit and loss account as in industry and commerce. It is not about dividing up the profits. The balance sheet in the public sector is public opinion and it is to that that the profession must address itself. That is why it would be a major mistake for nursing to allow the NHS to be broken up. Many nurses regard the existence of an NHS funded from taxation, comprehensive and free at the point of need as being the greatest social asset in the UK and an irreplaceable framework for the delivery of the best health care for all the people. They do not wish to see it divided and the public commitment to the service fragmented into commitment to whichever part is immediately required. If the public interest is diminished to the point where democratic pressure cannot secure change, then what avenue do nurses have except to resort to the sorts of political and industrial tactics employed by nurses in countries without a socialized health care system?

The existence of a comprehensive national health service is the hallmark of civilized society. It is also the major political framework within which nursing and its future is decided. Fragment and divide the health care system and nursing itself is fragmented and brutalized.

The nurses in the UK who join the RCN, and indeed the overwhelming majority who join other professional organizations, have made a pact with the public. They have given a guarantee that no matter how difficult the situation they will not withdraw their labour to pursue changes. That means that there must be an alternative avenue although it has hardly ever been effectively used. That alternative has existed since the inception of the NHS in 1948. The very character of a National Health Service controlled by national politicians lends itself to democratic political control and influence. That idea may seem distasteful to many people just as the idea of nurses being involved in politics is distasteful. By politics they usually mean partisan party politics. But it is possible to participate politically without being partisan. Political participation as an individual nurse and a member of an organization is infinitely preferable to the alternative of industrial action, inactivity and lack of reform or even the break up of the NHS.

Nursing faces a very difficult time ahead. In the frustration of the financial climate which is currently affecting the NHS and causing cycles of financial instability and temptation to imagine that a single act such as a strike will get results is very great. Yet the future of a service as large as the NHS will never be decided in that way. The debate may be delayed for a short while on particular issues, as happened with special duty payments in January 1988, but government will always eventually return to the issue on its terms unless the argument has been convincingly and politically won. There are no 'quick fixes' and industrial action by its very nature looks for a quick fix under the pressure of withdrawal of labour. What is at stake is a long-term pact with the public which in UK society is almost unique now to the nursing profession among public sector workers. That pact is maintained and pronounced upon by the public reflecting on the unquiet relationship which nursing has developed with government and all political parties. It is an unquiet relationship which should be maintained and which, if maintained, will break the cycles of disappointment which have characterized attempts to achieve reform and just pay levels for nurses for over three decades. There is no really effective alternative.

REFERENCES

Commission on Nursing Education (1985) *The Education of Nurses: a New Dispensation.* Royal College of Nursing, London (Chairman H. Judge).

Committee on Nursing (1972) *Report.* HMSO, London (Chairman A. Briggs).

Department of Health and Social Security. Committee of Inquiry into the Pay and Related Conditions of Service of Nurses and Midwives (1974) *Report.* HMSO, London (Chairman the Earl of Halsbury).

Department of Health and Social Security. Community Nursing Review (1986) *Neighbourhood Nursing – a Focus for Care. Report.* HMSO, London (Chairman J. Cumberlege).

Ministry of Health, Department of Health for Scotland and Ministry of Labour and National Service (1947) *Report of the Working Party on the Recruitment and Training of Nurses.* HMSO, London (Chairman R. Wood).

Ministry of Health and Scottish Home and Health Department (1966) *Report of the Committee on Senior Nursing Staff Structure.* HMSO, London (Chairman B. Salmon).

Parliament (1979) *Nurses, Midwives and Health Visitors Act.* HMSO, London.

Review Body for Nursing Staff, Midwives, Health Visitors and Professions Allied to Nursing (1987) *Fourth Report on Nursing Staff, Midwives and Health Visitors.* HMSO, London (Chairman J. Cleminson).

Royal College of Nursing (1964) *A Reform of Nursing Education: First Report of a Special Committee on Nursing Education.* RCN, London (Chairman H. Platt).

Standing Commission on Pay Comparability (1980) *Report No. 3: Nurse and Midwives.* HMSO, London (Chairman H.A. Clegg) (Cmnd. 7795).

Treasury (1987) *The Government's Expenditure Plans 1987–88 to 1989–90.* Volume 2. HMSO, London.

United Kingdom Central Council for Nursing, Midwifery and Health Visiting (1986) *Project 2000: a New Preparation for Practice.* UKCC, London.

7   The NHS: evolution or dissolution?

CHRISTINE HANCOCK

Colleges, hospitals and universities have grown larger than an earlier generation would have dreamed possible. Their budgets have grown even faster, yet everywhere they are in crisis. A generation or two ago their performance was taken for granted, today they are attacked on all sides for lack of performance.
Drucker (1977)

That could have been written in the United Kingdom in 1988 at the time of writing this chapter; yet it was written in the United States of America in 1977. It is hard to get a sense of perspective about the perceived and real state of crisis in the National Health Service (NHS) today in order to measure the problems and difficulties, especially the shortage of resources, against the very real achievements and progress. The NHS is often described as a wallowing bureaucracy, sucking in resources without real accountability. The figures of rising costs and increasing staff flow from politicians' mouths and journalists' pens. NHS staff numbers have doubled since 1948, increased by over 600000 in the past two decades. Can we demonstrate a better health service as a result, or are we just employing more people? These types of questions are being asked in more or less rational ways by many people.

Often the attacks on the NHS start in the House of Commons, from all sides, and particularly from the Public Accounts Committee and from the Parliamentary Select Committee on the Social Services. When any Secretary of State is questioned by these Committees he or she finds it difficult to be specific about the effect of Government policies, or indeed whether they were actually being pursued! He (since the days of Barbara Castle) finds it difficult to explain the very wide variations in the levels of provision in different parts of the country. He is certainly not able to say whether the NHS is efficient and whether the public is getting value for the money that they are spending.

The NHS was part of a number of social reforms introduced after the Second World War. In 1943, the Government accepted this particular reform which was designed to secure an improvement in the mental and physical health of the people and in the prevention, diagnosis and treatment of illness. Aneurin Bevan, the Health Minister at the time, said 'Society becomes more wholesome, more serene and spiritually more healthy if it knows that its citizens have at the back of their consciousness the knowledge that not only themselves, but also their fellows, have access when ill to the best that medical skill can provide'. The NHS has secured all-party support for 40 years; it has freed the people of this country from the fear of being unable to afford treatment for acute or chronic illness. Over 90% of health care in this country is provided through the NHS. Patients are free to seek and pay for care through the small private sector: doctors and other staff are free to work within the NHS or in the private sector, or both. Over 95% of total NHS expenditure is financed by central Government, 86% from general taxation, 11% from National Insurance contributions, and 3% from charges to patients for drugs and appliances (including spectacles) and dental treatment. Total expenditure on health care in this country is about 6% of our gross domestic product, whereas France and Germany spend 8–9% and the USA 11%. A key factor in the NHS is that it is free at the point of access. General Practitioners each provide general medical care to about 2000 people and access, when necessary, to specialists. There are problems of access to health care in Britain and these relate to geography, to social class, and to waiting times for certain conditions. Central London spends on average three times more per person per annum on health care compared with parts of the Midlands. Scotland and Northern Ireland spend more per person per annum than England, but have much worse mortality and morbidity rates. If the death rates of professional men were the same for all working men, it is estimated that 15 000 fewer working men would die in one year.

The NHS is popular with the British people as opinion polls show. One of its major problems, however, is that because demand is not limited by money, it is limited by waiting. Of patients who need treatment 45% are admitted within one month, but 6% wait over one year, and these average figures disguise very major problems in certain geographical areas and for certain conditions. Waiting times certainly encourage private practice which is particularly significant in certain medical conditions: for example, 25% of hip replacement in southern England and 50% of all abortions are undertaken in the private sector.

When a massive reorganization of the NHS was planned for 1974, many people were naive and optimistic enough to believe that this was planned in the interests of patients and that it was about bringing community health services and hospital services together. The Ministry produced some very smart charts which had the patient in large letters at the top of the family tree and the Minister of Health at the bottom! What the 1974 reorganization did do was to give to each Health Authority the full local responsibility for planning services for the local population: this was to make more true the promise of the NHS of equality of access to services right across the country. In particular, this was the first time that the famous teaching hospitals had specifically been asked to provide for a local population. One of the major features was that for the first time it brought many psychiatric and other long-stay hospitals into the same system of management as the general hospitals. That was extremely important in that it opened the eyes of, and indeed shocked, many senior staff, particularly nurses, when they saw the big difference in the standard which existed between the two sectors: different standards often in such matters as clothing and food. The main achievement of 1974 was to introduce District Management Teams, and a nurse was present on that Team, and, indeed, all other Management Teams where decisions about patients and patient care were made. However, the 1974 reorganization was introduced with very firm, rigid guidelines, and a further reorganization was introduced in 1982, because the 1974 system felt, and was, bureaucratic. It was also considered costly, although charges of high administrative costs in the NHS have always been made more on emotional than on factual grounds. In reorganizing, the assumption was yet again made that one structure would work for the whole country. The 1982 reorganization created more local Health Authorities, and provided a simpler structure. As in 1974, the introduction of the new management system coincided with a squeeze on resources, leading to much discussion about cuts.

> We trained hard but it seemed that every time we were beginning to form up into teams we would be reorganised. I was to learn later in life that we tend to meet any new situation by reorganising and a wonderful method it can be for creating the illusion of progress while producing confusion, inefficiency and demoralisation. (Caius Petronius, AD 66)

The 1982 reorganization had not had time to settle when a report was produced for the Government by an Inquiry Team chaired by Sir Roy Griffiths, the Managing Director of Sainsburys. The Inquiry Team published their report in 1983, in the form of recommendations and ten pages of background notes. That short report, followed by a DHSS circular (DHSS, 1984) produced change in the National Health Service which has been revolutionary rather than evolutionary. Early in the introduction of general management, the Royal College of Nursing ran one of its largest public campaigns alleging among other things that general managers did not know their coccyx from their humerus! Nurses were hurt, angered and shocked by the introduction of general management; similar reactions to those that patients feel with the sudden onset of illness or indeed the admission to a hospital. General management was introduced for two reasons: to simplify and improve getting things done and to improve the way that things are done. Many studies in nursing had shown that ward sisters in particular were concerned greatly over problems with support services which were nothing to do with nursing: laundry, catering, minor works and maintenance. Requisitions and complaints seemed just to disappear into thin air while taps continued to drip, light bulbs needed replacing and clean sheets were unobtainable on Sundays. Similarly, nurses are concerned, and certainly should be, when two patients are admitted and there is only one bed, when appointments systems lead to ten patients having the same appointment time; and when bereaved and grieving relatives are given their loved one's clothes and belongings in what looks like a dustbin liner. To provide appropriate nursing care nurses must share responsibility for the general standard of hygiene and nutrition provided to patients.

In his report Roy Griffiths stated that 'if Florence Nightingale were carrying her lamp through corridors of the NHS today, she would almost certainly be searching for the people in charge'. Others consider that Sir Roy is quite wrong. If Florence Nightingale were here today, *she* would be in charge and *she* would see that nurses were in charge wherever patients were being nursed and she would be horrified by the state of the hygiene, catering, ventilation and noise in many of our hospitals.

General management was introduced into the NHS to provide a coherent approach to health service management so that patients and others who used the Service were made aware at every point of contact with it that the system was organized to anticipate and meet their needs. General management was introduced to ensure clear decisions, tight control on spending, the appointment of the right staff, and it is about knowledge and understanding of the health needs of the population, and the care and treatment required by those who are sick or handicapped. General management should also be about leadership with which staff can identify and which encourages everyone's commitment and concern: it is this which will affect most the quality of care which patients receive.

Having authority, being in charge, getting things done, do not mean that one single dictatorial person orders everyone else around. Rather it means that people working together understand and share the same objective.

If general management means that things do actually get done in wards, hospitals, clinics and departments, and things are run smoothly and efficiently, then there can be no need for a further restructuring or reorganizing of the health service. If the introduction of general management has achieved improvements in the way services are delivered to patients, then it is hard to see why there is a need for further change.

There are three particular points within the Griffiths Report where the best insight into Roy Griffiths' own thinking comes out in his 'general observations'. First, 'that lack of general management process means that it is extremely difficult to achieve change'. Second, 'it cannot be said too often that the National Health Service is about delivery services to people'. Third, 'that there is little measurement of health output'.

Those working in health service management must recognize that there are many serious critics of the NHS and of the process of management. They include most people who look at the NHS from outside but, more seriously, many people working from within the NHS. That does not necessarily mean that the management structure is wrong; it may mean that too little time is spent examining how work is done and that the system is remote and confusing; it may mean that the NHS is an extremely complex and difficult business to manage. It may be that all three are important to some extent. As two of the three points mentioned will not change with a changed structure, it is not surprising that the structural changes made in the name of general management have not been the panacea that was anticipated. Similarly, the NHS should be careful of going blindly down the industrial path. It was surely the industrial problems of this country in the 1970s, when production fell by 15%, that caused the economic crisis which was felt so sharply in the NHS. Consideration should be given to the best private businesses. For they, in most cases, work with a degree of consensus. For example, Unilever, since Darcy Cooper's reforms of the 1930s, operates its large and complex multinational business by means of small committees. Look at the boards of successful businesses, and consider how many of them are run by managers with a generalist background, as opposed to managers with a very sound background in the business concerned. All eight of the executive directors of Imperial Chemical Industries have spent most of their careers in that company, although only one is a chemist. All six of the full-time directors of British Gas are 'gas people', and one could continue through other private businesses. The NHS needs to strengthen, not weaken, its management by using and developing the talented staff it has, particularly the doctors and nurses.

These points require careful consideration but the fact remains that Roy Griffiths is right. It has been extremely difficult to achieve change within the NHS. That is because of three things, which should be considered carefully. The first is not so much the lack of profit motive, but the lack of competition. If one does not like brand X cornflakes, it is very easy to buy brand Y. If one does not like what one sees or hears of one model of car, it is easy to choose from a range of others. Those decisions have a quick and immediate impact on the people running the businesses concerned. That does not happen in the NHS and more sophisticated management systems have to be developed to replace that simple mechanism which private businesses have. Second, many need to be reminded of that famous sign of Harry S. Truman which stated 'the buck stops here'. Before general management there was nothing in the NHS which ensured the buck stopped anywhere. Since general management, it is still possible to allow the buck to pass smoothly and easily ever upwards, so there still can be a feeling of exasperation that nobody is really in charge of the service.

The major change which Roy Griffiths brought to the NHS was not the introduction of general managers, but it was the general management process and, in particular, the requirement to consider the needs of patients and clients in the NHS, which is much more difficult and much more demanding than the marketing of many businesses. Before general management very few people would ever discuss marketing in terms of the NHS. Ted Levitt's 'Innovation in Marketing' makes interesting reading in the aftermath of the Griffiths Report, in particular this useful paragraph at the end of a chapter headed 'Management Myopia':

> Management must think of itself as providing customer-creating value satisfactions. It must push this idea (and everything it means and requires) into every nook and cranny of the organisation. It has to do this continuously, and with the kind of flair that excites and stimulates the people in it. Otherwise the business will be merely a series of pigeon-holed parts with no consolidating sense of purpose or direction. In short, the organisation must learn to think of itself, not as producing goods or services, but of finding customers, as doing the things that would make people want to do business with it. The Chief Executive has the inescapable responsibility for creating this environment, this viewpoint, this attitude, this aspiration. He must set the company's style, its direction and its goals. This means he had to know precisely where he himself wants to go, and he has to make sure the whole organisation is enthusiastically aware of where that is. This is the first requisite of leadership, for, unless you know where you are going, any road will take you there. If any road is alright, the Chief Executive might as well pack his attaché case and go fishing! If an organisation does not know or care where it is going, it does not need to advertise the fact with a ceremonial figurehead; everybody will notice it soon enough (Levitt 1962).

This comes back to the point already made: that everybody has noticed that the NHS does not always know where it is going. The major difference between the NHS and a commercial organization is that staff working in those successful businesses clearly know the objectives of the organization, and they have a commitment to fulfil those objectives. Within the NHS there are far too many people working with a variety of conflicting objectives, and it is rare to find the staff of a large hospital, let alone a whole health district, clearly sharing these objectives and committed to achieving them. Unless this point is recognized and accepted and careful consideration given both nationally and locally to how this can be changed, then general management will not have been enough, and it will not be possible to resist further demands for change.

The second of the general observations made by Roy Griffiths is so important that it should be quoted in full:

> It therefore cannot be said too often that the National Health Service is about delivering services to people. It is not about organising systems just for their own sake. In proposing the national health service in 1944, the Government declared that: 'the real need is to bring the country's full resources to bear upon reducing ill health, and promoting good health in all its citizens; and there is a danger of over organisation, of letting the machine designed to ensure a better service itself stifle the chance of 'getting on'. Our advice for management action is not directly about the nature of the services to provide its patients, but the driving force behind our advice is the concern to secure the best deal for patients and the community within available resources; the best value to the tax payer; and the best motivation for the staff. As a caring, quality service, the national health service has to balance the interests of the patient, the community, the tax payer, and the employees.

There are several specific areas where much more could be done about organizing the way in which the NHS is delivered to the people of this country. First, the question of the promotion of health: there is no question that within the health service lip service is still paid to the question of health promotion. How often can one walk into health care premises and find NHS staff smoking? The example of smoking is used, first because it is most visible and second because the statistical evidence about smoking is absolutely incontrovertible. There are, of course, other health promotion measures, and on the whole very little is done about these either. It is a serious matter if staff smoke at work, in wards or near patients, and the smell of a nurse or porter who has been smoking in a concealed rest room must be just as obvious to a patient as if they smoked in front of them, as indeed many of them do. It is like Store A claiming to sell good food but their staff all shop at Store B.

Second, the question of reception: when somebody comes into a hospital and into many primary health care centres, how often do they get a smile and a courteous and helpful reception? Matters such as this do not cost money.

Third, the question of waiting: real management effort has recently been put into abolishing inhuman and unacceptable ways of waiting for operations and in clinics and accident departments, but more could still be done to remove one of the major sources of dissatisfaction within the NHS. Some hospitals have worked systematically to reduce their waiting lists by a diary system, by day surgery, by more efficient use of theatres and by a shorter length of stay. More recently, central Government resources have provided new opportunities to work at particular waiting lists.

Fourth, the question of information: the sort of brochures and letters and signs that are around hospitals and clinics. If many of these were improved, perhaps it would not be long before the information which doctors and nurses give to patients also began to improve.

Finally, the hotel services: when somebody is ill at home, the sort of things that family and friends concentrate on is that the room they are in is clean and quiet, warm enough but not too hot and stuffy, that they have what they like to eat and drink, sometimes not a great quantity but often slightly unusual things at varying times of the day, and that they have the opportunity to sleep when they can. To paraphrase Roy Griffiths, if Florence Nightingale were carrying her lamp through the corridors of the NHS today, she would be most distressed by the state of the hotel services she found, and by the fact that many nurses no longer see these important areas of patient care as being their responsibility.

It is not necessary to look towards private businesses to find suitable models. One has only to look at the private health sector: there is much within the NHS that is done better than in the private sector, but whereas they treat patients as customers buying services, the NHS too often gives too little credit and respect.

A further observation from the Griffiths Report which needs to be highlighted is the question of measurement of health output. 'Businessmen have a keen sense of how well they are looking after their customers. Whether the national health service is meeting the needs of the patients and the community and can prove that it is doing so is open to question.' 95% of patients and clients in the NHS however are generally satisfied. There are many businesses which would like to be able to claim as much, but the areas of dissatisfaction for NHS patients and clients are known and too little effort is put into remedying them.

The question of output is important and there are a number of simple measures that could be worked with, while developing more sophisticated performance indicators. Does every hospital manager have available immediately details of clinics which were cancelled, of operating lists that were cancelled? Quite a small indicator of the major failure in service, but probably the one often only known to the person in the personnel department who could not find a locum, or to the theatre sister who knew that the anaesthetist was busy in the intensive care unit, or the ward sister who had inadvertently fed the only patient on the list that day.

The NHS is working in a very different environment from that of private organizations. In many areas it is an extremely successful organization, but there are large and significant areas of failure. The NHS is now being made to address itself seriously to those areas where the health service is not working, and where, if it blinds itself to the changes in patient expectation and indeed to staff expectation, it will see more and more exasperated attempts to change and restructure the organization.

Why is it now being suggested that the NHS may, or even should, be dissolved? Certainly the NHS is under attack, perhaps more than at any time since its introduction in 1948. Patients and others complain about long waiting lists, about waiting times in clinics, about doctors' poor communication, about large, bureaucratic, inefficient, unfriendly and often dirty hospitals, and overall about a lack of choice. Staff working in the service complain that Governments starve them of resources and when they work abroad receive much higher pay and see better equipment and facilities.

There is a good deal of debate concerning alternative sources of finance for the NHS. Most of the current anxieties, and indeed most of the proposals for change, relate to acute hospitals. Hospitals take the major part of the NHS financial resources; the high cost of medical technology affects the general hospitals; and when financial or other resources are short the publicity is greatest concerning acute hospital care. Some of the other parts of the NHS are for groups of people who cannot contribute significantly to the cost of their care.

On financing, one suggestion is to fund the NHS through national insurance contributions. A separate health contribution which appeared on payslips would, it is thought, make people aware of the true cost of the NHS. Health revenues could be linked automatically to earnings, and the rich could be allowed to contract out as they can from state earnings related pension schemes, although paying for a significant 'safety net'. However, this seems like a cosmetic device: people are not unaware of the true cost of the NHS. It would not introduce a direct link between the individual consuming health services and payment for them, nor would it be the only way of linking economic growth to NHS revenue; this could be achieved if there was the political will. Traditionally national insurance contributions are regressive and the effective tax burden on poorer people would rise, especially if rich people contracted out in large numbers. A special tax is traditionally disliked by the Treasury. It is not at all obvious that there would be a major change in the level of total funding in the NHS, even if the present reliance on general taxation was altered to earmarked taxation, local taxation or national health insurance for those able to pay.

Most western countries (apart from the United States) finance 80% or more of their health care from state finance, and even the USA pays for nearly half its health care this way. Similarly, it is rare in any country for patients to pay directly for health care at the time that they use it. What is different is that in Britain NHS finance comes from the Exchequer whereas in most other countries there is some kind of compulsory insurance. Britain spends at least 2% less of its national income on health care than comparable countries. However, the NHS is relatively cheap for two main reasons: the general practitioner acts as a barrier between patients and easy access to expensive hospitals; and pay is lower than in many other countries.

An interesting table in the annual financial report of one Health

Authority is the analysis of salary ranges. The 1985/6 report showed that just over 30% of the staff earned less than £5000; 69% earned less than £7500 and 90% earned less than £10,000. Whatever else may be said about motivation and commitment, it has to be acknowledged that these salaries are low and that this is a problem which has to be addressed. The problem, of course, is that even a small increase in NHS salaries and wages adds up to a very large bill, and public sector wage levels are an important element of any Government's economic policy. Commitment and motivation are a great asset but they should not be exploited. One way of making sure that the best use is made of human resources is to reduce the demotivating effect of low pay. Of course it is possible to show appreciation of people in many ways other than the rate of pay. Attitudes towards people can demonstrate their value, but society's values and appreciation are expressed in levels of pay. By rewarding people poorly a statement is being made about their value and society's view of them.

Another concern expressed by some relates to the small scale of the private health sector in Britain. Private health spending is only about 0.5% of gross domestic product in the United Kingdom, compared with nearly 2% in West Germany, nearly 3% in France, and about 6.5% in the USA. However, other countries have been reducing the relative size of their private health sectors in recent decades in recognition of their many inefficiencies. Administration which is popularly believed to be high in this country is around 20% in the USA compared with 5% for the NHS. Payment for private health care is usually on some sort of fee per item of service basis and doctors thus have a cash incentive to prescribe and to perform surgery. An American woman, for example, is three times more likely than a British woman to have a hysterectomy.

Diverting resources into a private sector is often wasteful and tinkering with the mechanism of financing the NHS does not seem as advisable as improving the operation of the present health service system. An American, Alain Enthoven, a professor from Stamford University in California, has looked at incentives to efficiency in health services management in the United Kingdom. His views were first published in the *Economist* in 1985 where his report was described as 'full, sympathetic and remarkable'. Professor Enthoven is best known for his proposal for an experimental internal market in the NHS. Health Authorities already buy and sell services between themselves and with the private sector. He has urged a large expansion of this kind of activity which is hampered by the lack of information on hospital costs. Each district would receive a budget based on its population and health needs but it would no longer expect to provide virtually all the services itself. Instead, it would buy and sell services from and to other districts and trade with the private sector. The hope would be that cost-efficient districts would expand their activities as resources flowed in from other areas, whereas the inefficient would be obliged to cut their physical provision of health care. The internal market is seen by its advocates as a way of reaping some of the supposed benefits of competitive private health without the unpleasant side effects. Access to care, for example, would remain independent of a person's income and districts would continue to have a blanket responsibility for the health of their communities. At the moment the DHSS resource allocation mechanism does not allow for direct cross-charging and movement of cash between Health Authorities. There is some attempt to compensate for cross boundary flows, but it is crude and works two years in arrears. So a region or district which attracts more patients can under present rules find itself losing money. As Enthoven himself noted, the best way to see how an internal market might work would be to experiment with it, perhaps in one region with all its districts.

For the past decade, service and resource strategy in the NHS has been directed at the objective of achieving equal access to health care services for equal needs. However, the debate about a market philosophy for the NHS has begun to undermine that original strategy and there is now some confusion about which approach has primacy. The goal has been to redistribute non-specialist hospital services so that they are normally provided close to where people live, to meet that objective of equal access for equal need. The directives of the Allocation Working Party (RAWP) have been used as the mechanism to achieve this goal. There are good reasons why this policy has survived so long and commands widespread political support. The majority of people who require hospital care are over 65, and the great majority obviously are ill or disabled in some way. Travelling becomes an additional burden, and distance diminishes the opportunity for social contact with family and friends, which influences recovery rates. While some younger and less-disabled people may be willing to travel if they have to, most people would prefer local accessible services. Better health care can usually be provided on a localized basis; few illnesses or disabilities can be treated in isolation; most need to be judged in the context of the individual's social, economic and physical environment. Hospital care is just one element of a whole range of voluntary and statutory services, which depend on personal contact and good communication if they are to be effectively coordinated. Such a localized policy is the basis of the objectives of the World Health Organization's *Health for All by the Year 2000* (World Health Organization, 1981).

Recently it has become increasingly clear that a policy which depends on shifting financial resources is neither an effective nor acceptable means of redistributing services, particularly where this involves real reductions in revenue allocation. Such enforced reduction in hospital capacity has led to faster patient throughput and rising waiting lists often with little impact on referral patterns. If redistribution of services is to be achieved, financial policies have to be backed up by strategies to influence referral patterns at source, or to relocate medical staff. In the meantime, a policy which depends on actual and visible cuts in services will always be hard to sell to local communities and staff of the health service, particularly in areas such as central London where media interest and attention is high. With an internal market, patients would effectively arrive with a 'dowry' and this would introduce an element of competition which could in turn drive down costs. However, this would require an explicit strategy to increase volume and specialization, to draw patients from a wider area, rather than to redistribute services so that they become more locally accessible. There is a danger that the idea of the internal market perpetuates a pattern and inhibits change. The attractive high technology work could be duplicated, and indeed diseconomies of scale can result if there is overprovision. Cold surgery is probably only 30% of hospitals' acute work and under 3% of the total NHS work. One suggested way to start an internal market might be to encourage GPs to refer to hospitals rather than to individual consultants, and allow the hospital then to deliver the service to the patient in a competitive way.

This leads to the other radical suggestion of the moment, which is some form of Health Maintenance Organization (HMOs). This concept which has developed in the USA, is designed to address the twin dilemmas of efficiency and choice. This plan was head-lined by *The Times* as 'GPs and their patients may be privatised'. Health maintenance organizations would operate as private companies which, for payment of a fixed monthly or annual premium, would provide a total service of health care for the patient over the year. These could be led by the general practition-ers, who would take with them their existing lists, together with a Government capitation fee. The organizations would be both insurers and providers of health care, possibly fixed around one hospital. In some versions, HMOs might own that hospital, or merely hire its services. Individual patients would not have to pay for their basic cover. That cost would be met by the Government's annual payment of a capitation fee based on so much per patient on the doctor's list, based largely on the age of each patient. The age groups would be banded according to the actuarial expect-ations of health care required for each group. The system would be sufficiently flexible to allow patients to pay for those things often thought to be extras, such as better food, private rooms and quicker attention. As private companies, the HMOs would have a considerable interest in private medicine to keep down their costs. In cities there would be a variety of competing organizations and patients would be able to choose which they wanted to join; in remote rural areas choice, as now, would be more limited. In the United States, HMOs grew up as a means of holding down the rapidly spiralling health costs, and there are now 393 serving more than 19 million people.

A British version of HMOs is currently being described as 'Managed Health Care Organizations' (MHCOs) which would separate the funding of health care from its provision and also exploit internal markets. Its advocates describe the NHS as a 'very large, very inefficient HMO' and by splitting it into small constitu-ent parts believe that the principles that have made HMOs success-ful in the US would apply in this country. MHCOs would combine the financing function of Health Authorities and Family Practi-tioner Committee (FPC) both of which would be abolished. The MHCO contract out the provision of services as an FPC does, but manage the use of delivery of health care like an HMO. A Health Care Financing Administration would finance HMCOs on a capitation basis according to the population which they served. Funding would then be based on a similar criteria to that of

RAWP. MHCOs would contract with local hospitals and with private hospitals to provide services. Both GPs and hospital consultants would be given much tighter contracts than at present, and their performance would be monitored more intensely. According to the proponents of MHCOs they would have a great advantage of flexibility and choice; patients would be free to change their MHCO and Government funding would travel with them. It is envisaged that one MHCO would serve populations of between 100000 and 200000, less than the size of the average health district now. The system would certainly still operate as a health service funded from general taxation, free at the point of delivery to all regardless of need. However, patients would have the right to opt out and seek private care. The MHCO would also hold contracts with hospitals to provide a fixed number of bed days a year for certain specialties. For example, the MHCO might have a contract with two hospitals to provide hip operations and two hospitals for maternity services. The MHCO would choose the hospital depending on rates and quality of service, which would be determined by the views of patients and by an extensive system of peer review. The MHCOs would be able to purchase services from either the public or private sector from any part of the country under an internal market system. Their local MHCO would not necessarily be responsible for providing their care, only funding it.

There are a number of studies taking place on the issue of alternative methods of funding the NHS. The purpose of these studies undoubtedly varies. In some cases the search is to find easy ways of raising more money for the NHS, ways that perhaps will inflict less pain on the tax payer. Others are looking for more accountability from the providers of health services to the consumer and the general public; a firmer link between the user and the provider. Others are looking for a more competitive approach between Authorities and perhaps a switch in balance in the provision of services between the NHS and the private sector. Whatever the purpose, much greater knowledge is needed on how the service is presently using the resources it already has available. There is no point in either just pumping more and more money into the health services or of proposing radical and dramatic structural change without a clearer understanding of how well money is being used now — the standards, type and quality of services being provided. More detailed information on the case mix that hospitals are already treating and their cost is essential before furthering some of the options being discussed, e.g. the internal market model; greater privatization. It is not realistic to attempt to specify contracts to let services to the private sector without greater information on case mix and costs. Also, in this context, improved accountability of the service to the public is crucial and some of the proposals for change would clearly help in this.

But in pursuing efficiency the NHS dare not forget quality and choice. Health Authorities are also actively trying to find out how the services are perceived by patients and how well they meet what is required. Many are using survey methods of one kind or another, and many are providing staff with the encouragement to identify, analyse and resolve problems. The health service has to concentrate attention on access, choice, information and redress. Access to services is obviously the crucial first stage for the potential consumer, and the Black Report (DHSS, 1980) showed continuing inequalities in this. Choice means that professionals have to deliver care in ways which satisfy their patients. Changes in clinical practice are slowly occurring as a result of consumer pressure, pressure which might have been unthinkable ten or twenty years ago, and less common in this country than in others. Examples of this are the more varied choices now offered to women in childbirth and the trend away from mastectomy as a means of treating breast cancer – both measures generated in large measure by consumers themselves.

Access to quality services and the opportunity to choose between services have to be supported with useful information with which to make that choice and the power to seek redress if things go wrong. Is there an inherent conflict between efficiency and effectiveness in health care; between quantity and quality? The debates about the future shape of the Health Services need to consider both audiences: the taxpayer who foots the bill and the patient who requires the treatment. Those providing health care, whether public or private, have a responsibility not only to make the most cost effective use of resources but to ensure that the provision actually meets what people want.

In the search for a radical solution to the current problems of the NHS, and the use of words such as 'dissolution', there is a very real danger of understating the considerable achievements and potential of the NHS. The private sector is small in this country in relation to the NHS and the dangers of copying the United States with unregulated growth, increased costs, but no improved health, seems unlikely to be considered seriously by policy makers. It is likely that more and more people will use both the NHS and private health care, rather than one or the other, and that will no doubt have a profound effect on both.

In the current debate on the 'crisis of the National Health Service' there must be cause for concern that the NHS itself allows the use of crisis in such general terms. Almost all commentators speak of the need for more resources; the debate is only about the source and use of those resources. Yet much of the debate seems to be questioning more fundamentals than just funding, and equally obscuring other serious issues. There remains within the NHS a lack of a confident corporate commitment to a future health service which may in part be inspired by political commentators challenging its very foundations but increasingly seems to be challenging those foundations more strongly than any of the commentators. The very complexity of health care and of managing health systems must be a contributory factor to that but so also is a bureaucratic system which despite general management continues to have real difficulty in feeling that locally there is autonomy and choices which can be made and decisions implemented. These are the issues which need to be addressed.

The crisis of the NHS is not the one about which so much is being written and debated so much as the need to respond to the health care needs of the growing number of elderly people; the need to have health care systems which make the best use of the dwindling numbers of available staff and the need to have a health care system which improves the health outcome measures of the people in this country to resemble more closely those of many of our European neighbours. These are the crises which endanger the NHS more than many of those currently being debated. The reality of the NHS may be that one 'would not start from here' but for few will there ever be the opportunity to devise a new system from a fresh start. Evolution based on the strength of the present NHS must be the only sensible way forward and the NHS itself across all political views and vested interests should be united in saying this to politicians of all parties. The political management of the NHS needs to create a culture and reward system that guides the thousands of decisions which are made each day in the direction of better quality care and service at reduced costs. This is where the present NHS structure is weakest. It relies too heavily on dedication and idealism. It often seems to be propelled by the conflicting interests of different provider groups and it offers few positive incentives to do a better job for the people who will pay for their health care under any system.

Finally, to quote from one of the gurus of the current debate, Professor Alain Enthoven:

> Public policy and responsible politicians should seek to create an environment for the NHS that is hospitable quality-improving and efficiency-improving change. There is a need to work at loosening up the system so that new things can be tried, and so that successful innovations can be spread. Opportunities for constructive change should be nurtured, not politicised or otherwise abused. (Enthoven, 1985)

REFERENCES

Department of Health and Social Security (1980) *Inequalities in health: report of a research working group.* DHSS, London (Chairman Sir D. Black).

Department of Health and Social Security (1984) *Implementation of the NHS management inquiry report.* DHSS, London (HC(84)13).

Drucker, P. (1977) *Management.* Harpers College Press, New York.

Enthoven, A.C. (1985) *Reflections on the Management of the National Health Service: an American Looks at Incentives to Efficiency in Health Services Management in the UK.* Nuffield Provincial Hospitals Trust, London.

Gloucester Health Authority (1986) *Annual Financial Report 1985–86.* GHA, Gloucester.

Levitt, T. (1962) *Innovations in Marketing.* McGraw-Hill, Maidenhead.

NHS Management Inquiry Team (1983) *NHS Management Inquiry: (letter to the Secretary of State).* The Team, London (Team leader E.R. Griffiths).

World Health Organization (1981) *Health for all by the year 2000.* WHO, Geneva.

8 Nursing in the future: a cause for concern

JANE ROBINSON

This chapter is about the marginalization of nursing care: in simpler terms, how can the activities and concerns of half a million waged nurses, and many more unpaid carers, remain largely invisible in the policy arena? The following quotations, which are concerned with the competing pressures upon public health policy makers and managers, the ambivalence among waged nurses about the nature of their role, and the strain upon un-numbered, unpaid women who care invisibly within the home, sum up part of the dilemma:

> By next year, we're going to have to go for reductions in the service, not just holding things steady. And on top of this, of course, there is pressure for new services, for cervical screening and breast screening and hip replacement and AIDS. At the end of the day, it's a question of the sort of society we want. Having to make choices when provision is being reduced is extremely divisive . . . but that is the road we are being pushed towards. The potential for doing nothing for the old, the mentally ill and the socially useless is tremendous.
>
> District General Manager (DGM)
> (Strong and Robinson, 1988)

Society has to decide what sort of nurses it wants. If it wants nurses to bathe us and make us comfortable, that's not a problem. We still have loads of applications for Enrolled Nurses. But if society wants a practitioner with some science and research knowledge then things will have to change. If society wants intelligent nurses things can't go on for long like this. People with 5 'O' levels aren't going to tolerate the way they're treated now. Society has changed . . . we're becoming more materialistic. These are the criteria by which people judge things. Nurses are a lot more realistic than they once were.'

Director of Nurse Education (DNE)
(Strong and Robinson, 1988)

First of all, in the morning Michael's got to be got up and dressed and fed and toileted, and you know he's got to be held on the toilet – you can't leave him. It's a couple of hours, really. And you can't do anything else while you're feeding him. If you turn round, it's spat out. It's a couple of hours getting him ready for school. And then when he comes home at half past three your time is devoted to him. Someone has to be there. And when he goes to bed you're constantly turning him. He has to be turned so many times before he goes to sleep. And he can be sick three times in the night . . .

Mother of 15 year old,
quadriplegic spastic boy
(Baldwin and Glendinning, 1983)

Susan Reverby (1987) in her recent synthetic history of American nursing probably expresses the problem best of all:

> . . . a crucial dilemma in contemporary (American) nursing (is) the order to care in a society that refuses to value caring . . . nursing is a form of labor shaped by the obligation to care. But its history, and ultimately its identity, cannot be understood unless the bond that has wedded it to womanhood is also unravelled and revealed.

This chapter is also, therefore, about nursing as caring, and about caring as a women's issue, and how both are pushed to the margins in the economic debates about health care.

Why should society refuse to value caring? First, presumably, because caring is cheap. It is something which half the population (namely women) are expected to do intuitively – why pay for caring if you have a mother, or a wife, who will do it for nothing? Second, caring has a dual meaning. Despite its ubiquity, caring does not exist in a free market. Instead, the obligation to care is dependent on a caste type hierarchy of gender relationships and women's socialization, as Graham (1985) puts it 'caring touches simultaneously on who you are and what you do.' Caring is work therefore as well as identity. Caring is also shaped, however, by the context in which it is practised. 'Particular circumstances, ideologies, and power relations . . . create the conditions under which caring can occur, the forms it will take, and the consequences it will have for those who do it.' (Reverby, 1987)

Current circumstances suggest that in the present context those conditions for caring may be changing. Variations in the demand and supply of women's labour suggest for instance that the price of caring is about to rise. Yet something so marginal, so hard to define, slips through our fingers just as we think that we can hold it firmly in our grasp. There is a need to explore the concept further, to understand the marginalization of caring a little better.

Both general and economic dictionary definitions of the term marginalization are relevant to the discussion here; first, as something close to the lower limit of qualification, acceptability or function, and, second, as the lower limit beyond which economic activity cannot be conducted under normal conditions. Exploration of the marginalization of nursing care will be considered here from predominantly feminist and economic perspectives. These two main sections are written sequentially. Ultimately, however, theoretical constructions will have to be developed which subsume these and other aspects of care in order to understand waged nursing's position in a general caring structure. The final section considers whether our assumptions about a gendered division of labour in caring have been, or will continue to be valid in future. If this chapter does nothing more than to set out an agenda and stimulate debate among those who are also feeling their way towards these issues, then it will have achieved its main intention.

THE BACKGROUND

Despite contemporary recognition by nurses that care is central to nursing, that it contains emotional and practical components as well as formal knowledge and skill, and that waged nursing care is complementary in certain specific circumstances to informal, unpaid caring (Henderson, 1966; Leininger, 1981, 1984; Kitson, 1987; RCN, 1987), developing the conceptual framework which can encompass adequately the relationships between nursing as caring in both the public and domestic domains is still some distance away. Tackling this issue is crucial as demographic change generates policy concerns in relation both to an ageing population, and to a shortage of recruits to nursing. These problems bring in train potentially loaded questions about the justification for various forms of skill mix in waged nursing care (not just in hospital, but in new types of residential provision and in the home); the relationship of paid to unpaid carers; the length and type of education and training needed for the providers of all forms of care; and, ultimately, how, why and whether women should be reimbursed for the care of sick and dependent relatives in the domestic domain (Land, 1982; Rimmer, 1983; Walker, 1983; Groves and Finch, 1983).

Without more understanding of these sensitive issues satisfactory explanations will never be gained as to why caring as women's work is marginalized, and why waged nursing care is usually at the bottom of the formal health policy agendas.

WAGED NURSING

Waged nursing today is in a highly ambiguous position. The size of the labour force is vast – 3% of all public expenditure (National Audit Office, 1985). There are approximately 550 000 nurses, midwives and health visitors currently on the United Kingdom Central Council's (UKCC) register. Not a day passes at present without the media devoting space to nursing issues, notably in terms of labour shortages and pay. Nursing in 1989 probably has a higher public profile than at any other time in the twentieth century, and with the greater political awareness of its professional organizations (Clay, 1987) nurses are learning fast how to use this situation to their advantage.

Yet, at the same time, one consistent and key factor has emerged from the findings of the Nursing Policy Studies Centre's (NPSC) empirical research into the management of nursing after

Griffiths (NHS Management Inquiry Team, 1983) (Robinson and Strong, 1987; Strong and Robinson, 1988) – that is the invisibility of most nursing issues to everyone except nurses. Despite the impressive statistics there remains the most profound ignorance amongst non-nurses about many nursing concerns and most nursing practice. In other words, despite the efforts which nurses themselves have made over the past two decades in reflecting on the nature of, and research into, nursing issues, the results appear to have made virtually no impact on others. It has been found that the majority of doctors and general managers alike had very little insight into current developments within nursing. Nurses themselves often seem, in turn, defensively unable to see their work within any broader policy context, and this mutual myopia has come to be described as the 'Black Hole of Nursing'. It sometimes appears, therefore, that those on the inside of nursing and those on the outside inhabit two different worlds, each holding both correct and incorrect perceptions of the other. Problems such as the tension between bureaucracy and humanity are widely known to both, but possible solutions are not. The subject is not usually even on the agenda for discussion.

In view of nursing's past history, this background is not at all surprising. A brief review of the literature on nursing a hundred years ago reveals similar contemporary concerns with recruitment and retention (Maggs, 1983), wages (Carpenter, 1980), education, registration and internal conflicts within the profession (Donnison, 1977; White, 1978). Small wonder then if nurses come to view the impending demographic crisis simply as an unprecedented policy ace with which to bargain over a number of key policy issues, a position summed up recently in the *Independent* newspaper; 'A dilemma for the health service could become the biggest boost to women workers since the war as competition for their skills forces employers to take their particular needs into account' (Phillips, 1987).

Yet it is the very timelessness of these substantive issues together with the continued obscurity of the conceptual problems surrounding nursing as caring which should give nurses cause for concern. If future progress is determined solely by nurses' scarcity, then it has to be remembered that nurses have been in short supply before, and nothing much has changed in the past. Governments have an uncanny knack of coming up with low-cost solutions which leave the basic problems untouched. That is why it seems to be so important to tease out some of the underlying structural issues which impact on nursing. Such activity lies at the basis of the policy studies enterprise, and it is through this that one hopes to gain a deeper insight into the nursing enigma.

Policy studies involves not just the gathering of facts about an issue, but also the analysis of how and why some issues get selected as a serious problem for public concern while others, potentially no less important, are neglected (Bachrach and Baratz, 1962). The how and why crucially concern matters of power and influence (Lukes, 1986). The anomaly of nursing is why, with little of either, on the one hand it has suddenly become a matter of such huge concern and on the other, is so little understood.

How can this unchanging situation be explained and is it possible that fresh insights could help to lead to change? If so, waged nurses have to broaden their perspective in order to understand the structures and beliefs that oppress all women, albeit with different costs and benefits to certain individuals. The idea to be developed here is the notion that nursing is an essentially marginal activity. Marginal, that is, both to the major policy concerns of the public domain of waged labour, and also of the domestic domain of non-waged work. The search begins with sources associated with, but surprisingly rarely directly related to waged nursing, feminist theory and health economics. In this way some useful connections may be made which could begin to help us to understand the problems more clearly.

WOMEN'S CARING WORK: MARGINALIZATION AND GENDER

Reading the feminist literature on lay carers, there are good conceptual grounds for treating both paid and unpaid caring labour analytically in the same way, that is as it appears to be ubiquitously perceived – as women's work, and therefore marginal to the major, public policy concerns of man. Unfortunately, this somewhat simple analytical device has been obscured by the fact that, in general, the larger parts of the two groups who have studied caring as fundamental to nursing (feminist theorists and nurses themselves) have, in pursuing their particular interests, failed to take the activity seriously as a unified whole. Olesen and Lewin (1985) acknowledge the feminist omission, pointing out that 'because of the unconscious incorporation of certain misogynist biases into even feminist thought, some critical topics – notably nursing – were largely overlooked by women's health researchers' (Lewin, 1977).

It is a commonplace that waged nursing is women's work – the term mother surrogate is not unusual (Schulman, 1958, 1972; Wilson, 1971; Brown, 1975; Bullough, 1975) and iconoclasts freely blame Florence Nightingale for setting in stone the sub-ordination of female nurses to male doctors (Gamarnikow, 1978; Whittaker and Olesen, 1964; Smith, 1982; Stacey, 1987). Never-theless, despite the recognition that care is central to waged nursing which fills, when necessary, some gap in the lay care situation, a conceptual framework which adequately encompasses care in both the public and domestic domains is still lacking.

In treating caring (*qua* nursing) separately in this way both groups have failed to address the common elements of knowledge and skill, and their repression as policy issues, found in both arenas. Stacey (1981) who is a notable exception, defines the terms of reference:

> I use the terms public and private or domestic domain to distin-guish two areas of action. They have nothing to do with the private and public sectors of industry . . . The private domain is the domain of the home, where social relations are based on family and kin . . . The public domain includes government and the market place. "The public sphere is that sphere in which 'history' is made. But the public sphere is the sphere of male activity. Domestic activity becomes relegated to the private sphere, and is mediated to the public sphere by men who move between both. Women have a place only in the private sphere" (Smith, 1974)

Although, historically, there has always been some regulation of family life by external institutions – notably the state or the church – some feminists have claimed that the process of industrialization has accelerated and intensified this situation. They argue that a characteristic of the modern industrialized world is the separation of the domestic from the public, which means in turn that the domain to which women commit a large part of their energy, expertise and emotion distinguishes it as being private and therefore beyond political analysis. Women's activities have therefore been dominated and subordinated by this exclusion (Graham, 1979, 1985; Finch and Groves, 1983; Evans, 1986; Ungerson, 1987).

Stacey (1981) points out that nursing was one of the human services translated from the late nineteenth century onwards from the private to the public domain, and therefore into the waged sector. This had two major consequences for the marginalization of nursing.

First, and perhaps currently of least concern to nurses but the matter to which most feminists direct their attention, is the invasion of the private domain by experts and representatives of the state. Stacey (1981) observes:

> The ability of the unwaged workers, parents and especially mothers, to perform their tasks and indeed their entire social roles without expert guidance has increasingly been called into question (Graham, 1979) . . .
> No longer are we allowed to believe that anything 'just comes naturally', except perhaps that it is still 'natural' for women to stay at home to rear the children they have borne and to do the associated service tasks.

The development of a waged welfare sector has led, so it is argued, to the deskilling of the women who remain at home, or, at least, to the devaluing of their intuitive and experientially learned caring skills. Some of these very acts of deskilling or devaluing may be carried out by midwives, nurses and health visitors who have become the waged experts in the public domain. The argument is, of course, grossly oversimplified. A great deal of 'scientific' advice from doctors as well as nurses is of the 'what every mother knows' variety. Indeed, it seems that what may really matter is the way in which advice is structured and given (Robinson, 1982). Nevertheless the 'social control' argument has had a powerful impact as a range of consumer surveys testify.

The second consequence is one which most feminists ignore, or at least treat simply as the male medical ascendancy over female healers (Pascall, 1986). That is, the transfer to the public domain of some of those very caring functions, claimed to be intuitive, or experientially learned in the private domain, which are then deemed by policy makers, managers and doctors to be of such low skill that they are not worthy of status, research or educational development.

Waged nursing finds itself, therefore, in a double bind. Translated to the public domain it is still perceived as women's work for which no special attributes, education or research is required. Nursing as 'tender loving care' encapsulates the prevailing attitudes. Yet, when nurses are encouraged as a matter of policy to treat their skills as a valuable educational resource for preventive and health promotion activities (often with clients in the private domain) then they are perceived by many of the recipients of their attention as agents of social control (Dean and Boulton, 1980). Paradoxically, the abhorrence of the infringement of individual liberty which lies at the heart of this rejection is shared not only by feminists but also by politicians of both right and left persuasions. Paid nurses, it seems, can never win.

Thus nursing is seen as women's work marginalized in two ways. Feminists, in concentrating on high quality unpaid care in the domestic domain draw attention to the reproduction of capital and patriarchal social relations, through the unwaged labour of women in the home. Nursing as caring is seen here to be marginalized because the personal is not believed by men to be political. Waged nursing on the other hand is marginalized both by the women who argue the case for the informal carers, and also by the men who control the health sector in the public domain. The women who provide the care in both situations not only find themselves without any substantial power base – they are also potentially divided against each other.

Can this situation be explained? It appears that not much theoretical development has taken place since Stacey (1981) claimed that:

> There appear to be two separate accounts . . . one that it all began with Adam Smith and the other that it all began with Adam and Eve . . .
> The problem arises because we lack a conceptual framework, let alone a theory with any explanatory power, which will permit us to analyse paid and unpaid labour . . . within one notion of the division of labour; which can encompass the domestic arena of Adam and Eve as well as the industry of Adam Smith.

Stacey's introduction of Adam Smith and his association with the market economy suggests that progress is unlikely to be made in understanding the contradictions inherent in women's caring roles until their economic aspects are more thoroughly investigated. If, for social and demographic reasons the pending scarcity of women's labour is likely to become permanent, then an assessment of its economic value seems overdue. The neglect of any serious attention to caring work by most of the social sciences is seen at perhaps its most extreme in health economics. This particular omission will be discussed in the second half of the chapter. Graham (1985), however, referring to this question of disciplinary blindness (and paradoxically for the purposes of this chapter) regrets that medical sociology and social policy have both been concerned almost entirely with the social relationships which operate within the waged sector of care, that is in medicine and in the social services. She claims that as a result study of the informal sector is restricted to its place as a site for consumption rather than the production of services. Yet waged nursing has, by and large, also been excluded from this public welfare sector analysis. Medical sociology has paid relatively little attention to nursing other than in its relationship to the process of male domination of professionalized health care. Nursing, as ubiquitous caring work which straddles both domains, has been largely ignored.

Some exceptions do exist. Analysts writing on the social services in particular have begun, at least, to address the question of 'whose labour, provided where?' Finch (1984), for example, draws out the complex factors operating in the domiciliary and residential fields of care. She reluctantly concludes that there are no easy or obvious solutions to the 'impasse of sexual divisions' in caring. If existing policies for 'Community Care' exploit women's unpaid labour, then realistic alternatives would do exactly the same. Eventually, she gives a cautious vote in the direction of residential care, pointing to its obvious limitations, but also acknowledging that it would give recognition to the fact that 'caring is labour, and in a wage economy should be paid as such'.

Two international health and social policy texts specifically consider caring and women's work in the light of future health care and demographic demands upon national and international policy making. Both assert that the inflationary spiral of health care costs will only be contained, and future needs met, through governments recognizing that 'all policy is care policy' (Secretariat for Futures Studies, 1984).

Pizurki, *et al.* (1987) consider women's role in relation to the World Health Organization strategy for Health for All (HFA) which includes community participation, multisectoral and international collaboration, and health care systems based on primary health care. These policies involve changes in the perceptions and roles of formal and informal carers, including the place of nursing, and of other female health care professionals. Adam (1987) (in reviewing Pizurki *et al*, 1987) points out, however, just how deeply ingrained gender differences in health care really are. In acknowledging the book's value she also sums up the scale of the difficulties:

> . . .in highlighting what for me is the major problem – how to consider the needs of women informal carers (who are themselves a hugely varied group), alongside low paid health workers, health professionals, and the few women health providers with high status and high incomes.
>
> I fully support the present initiatives to ensure that the NHS is an 'equal opportunities employer' and to address the special needs of women in management. But we are fooling ourselves if we think that these will, of themselves, change fundamentally the position of women health providers.
>
> Wider changes are required – for example, to enable men to develop their role as informal health providers, to support senior women health workers in retaining and expressing their woman-ness, and to continue to challenge the established professional and gender power hierarchies within the formal health-care system.

To consider caring as a unified whole is, of course, very difficult. For example, despite the many, as yet, unsubstantiated claims which are being made for the benefits of de-institutionalization, many are still wildly ignorant about the long-term impact of such policies. Further, current concern with demographic issues is only one aspect of a constantly shifting historical scene in patterns of health and disease and of their associated forms of service provision. Not only is there a conceptual and practical dichotomy between the private and public domains but also, within the latter, there are many divided and vested interests. Brief reflection on the distinction between caring provided by the health service on the one hand, and social services on the other, immediately throws up the many tensions which can be found between different public sector departments and different professional groups in caring, for example, for the victims of child abuse (Dingwall, Eekelaar and Murray, 1983) or the mentally handicapped. If there is an unsettled problem in the health service of overlap with social services, social work at present is just as uncertain of its future as nursing.

It is hard, even within NHS nursing alone, to develop theoretically based strategies for care which encompass both skilled and unskilled labour. Professional organizations represent the interests of qualified nurses and pre-credential students. The health service trade unions, in general, represent unqualified carers. Nursing policy, for the majority of qualified nurses, means no more than that – policy relating to nurses holding statutory qualifications. The anxieties raised by going beyond that definition can be found in the discussions of the statutory bodies over their involvement in the preparation of a new breed of support worker. Reverby (1987), in the history cited at the beginning of this chapter, sees for example that the 'shop floor' culture which gave American working-class nurses solidarity with other working groups was so much in conflict with the professionalizing aspirations of their upper class leaders that the possibility of internal, occupational cohesion within nursing was seriously reduced. In Britain, Carpenter (1978, 1980) writing on asylum nursing, and on nursing managerialism after Salmon carries similar messages. This argument, too, is in danger of being over-simplified. The way in which occupation determines social class for men does not apply for women. Qualified nurses may all be classified as Social Class II by the Registrar General, but as members of a women's occupation nurses, like secretaries, are drawn from a broad spectrum of social backgrounds. Status divisions in such a vast labour force are inevitable, and very complex. What is needed now is a serious analysis of how such divisions are structured, and to what extent they act dysfunctionally both to the organization and to individuals.

Policies relating to nursing as caring, unlike medicine with its tight professional boundaries, are usually considered, therefore, in fragmented and unequal ways. No study has yet confronted, for example, the persistent catch-22 situation of how nurses and governments operating in real time dimensions control the labour consequences of supplier-led demand for health care. The practical difficulties of managing nursing in the face of the medical profession's power to shape the service is illustrated by the following quotation from a Chief Nurse Adviser:

> . . .the real problem over there is that there are far too many doctors and far too many sub-speciality doctors, some of whom have only got half a dozen beds . . . and they all want to expand. If you take university appointments into account, on Floor 3 there are almost as many doctors as there are nurses! (Robinson and Strong, 1987)

Indeed, Pizurki *et al.* (1987) admit that:

> Of all professions subject to sex-role stereotyping, nursing seems the most severely handicapped in that nurses are doubly conditioned into playing a subservient role: first by society generally, and secondly by the medical establishment.

It is this seemingly intractable dependence of waged nursing on medically led developments, and the possible consequences in terms of equity in health care which will be considered now.

THE ECONOMICS OF NURSING: WHAT FORMS OF CARING ARE COST EFFECTIVE?

The short answer to this question is, of course, that this is unknown. A recent article (Delamothe, 1988) said of facts about nursing:

> It is surprising that so little is known about any resource, human or otherwise, which is worth so much. Information about the numbers moving into and out of nursing and their reasons for doing so is hard to come by. The most recent nurses' review body had cause to complain: 'The lack of comprehensive and up-to-date data has been particularly regrettable this year. The anecdotal material which has reached us from various sources strongly suggests that there have been significant changes recently in the manpower situation, but there are no statistics to give a reliable picture of what has been happening'. (Review Body for Nursing Staff, Midwives, Health Visitors, and Professionals Allied to Medicine, 1987).

This absence of up to date, appropriate and relevant data is not, from a policy analysis perspective, surprising. Until the present nursing 'crisis' the shortage of nurses could always be remedied by policies which encouraged some of the vast reservoir of women outside waged health care to come inside, and to nurse. The recruitment of VADs during the First World War, and the introduction of second-level assistant nurse training during the second, are both cases in point. There was no need, therefore, to keep accurate and up to date statistics for a workforce that could always be replenished from somewhere. In 1988, probably for the first time, this situation no longer exists. Demographic change and alternative career opportunities for women have resulted in an unprecedented and dramatic shift of waged nursing onto the policy agenda. The historically invisible policy issue has become, almost overnight, highly visible. That the data needed to define the scale of the problem do not exist is merely a reflection of nursing's past marginal policy position.

Nowhere is the invisibility of nursing issues more remarkable than in health economics. Despite the size of the workforce and the cost of caring in general, it is possible to look through contemporary texts and discover that nursing, caring, and labour costs are not even indexed. Gray (1987), in a broad search of the literature, identified only 200 serious nursing economics references, 90% of which originated in the USA.

The invisibility of nursing costs and therefore their marginalization from the health care priorities debates became apparent on reading three papers on Diagnostic Related Groupings (DRGs) (Kalisch and Kalisch, 1985; Milio, 1985; Melosh, 1986). It appears that where DRGs are used in the USA nursing costs are merely collapsed into the daily room rate together with other 'overheads'. American nurses have therefore challenged the validity of the DRG indicator as an adequate predictor of the real costs of care. The three authors also identify other direct and indirect effects of DRGs, for example, the opportunity they provide for enhancing the professional power and status for some nurses whilst impoverishing others, and the possible costs and benefits for patients. The point here is that even when using a sophisticated system such as DRGs nursing costs remain hidden, and therefore are not amenable to independent comparison and evaluation.

The relative costs of nursing in various health care contexts is a policy issue to which most nurses in Britain probably pay little attention. Yet it is a crucial component in debates about the most effective deployment of scarce nursing skills. Despite, for example, the many assertions which are being made in the North American literature that an all-qualified nursing staff is the most efficient in terms of productivity, which includes higher competence levels, lower wastage rates, less time spent in supervising unskilled staff, Gray (1987) identified few methodologically sound studies. In the United Kingdom Pearson (1987) at Oxford and Burford not only supports the North American view, but also argues the case for greater autonomy of the nursing role. This challenge contains the potential for nurses to determine, independently of medicine, not only their efficiency, but also the most effective deployment of nursing skills. Part of this efficiency is claimed to arise from the more effective use of unqualified staff in supporting the qualified; that is, arguing not just for greater **technical efficiency**, where the inputs of nursing care produce output at lowest possible opportunity cost, but also for **allocative efficiency**, which adds the notion of **effectiveness** (an optimal combination of outputs produced by means of the most technically efficient combination of inputs) (Gray, 1987).

Such research is, as yet, still in a relatively early development stage. It is fraught with methodological difficulties, and has not yet seriously addressed the *a priori* assumption that different skill mixes work differently in different situations. A dozen major studies are required with highly significant results before the claims can be effectively substantiated. Nevertheless, these are the arguments and techniques which health economists are already applying, in theory at least, to medical care. Identifying, and placing a value upon a defined output in relation to specific health care inputs lies at the basis of Quality Adjusted Life Years (QALYs). Whilst yet in an experimental stage, QALYs offer the possibility of placing a monetary value upon the production, through a medical intervention, of one year of life at full quality (Maynard, 1987).

Preliminary work (Williams, 1987a, pages 9 and 10) suggests, for example, that the following costs would be incurred for the associated interventions:

Hospital haemodialysis	£15000 per QALY gained
Heart transplantation	£8000 per QALY gained

Kidney transplantation	£3500	per QALY gained
Coronary artery bypass grafting	£2000	per QALY gained
Hip replacement	£750	per QALY gained
GP trying to persuade every smoker who visits them to give up	£200	per QALY gained

There are, of course, profound moral and ethical arguments about the use of QALYs. Should medical intervention ever be graded in this way? Should medical care always be freely available regardless of cost? If financial resources are finite, how should care be allocated – by ability to pay, or by social prestige, age, sex, colour?

Quality adjusted life years do help to concentrate the mind, however, on the apparently infinite possibilities for medical expansion set against the finite availability of financial resources, and there are lessons here for nurses, for the costs of nursing care are, as yet, not made explicit in such analyses. Do nurses, for example, have a right to know exactly what proportion of the nursing budget is devoted to specific medical techniques? If the answer to that question is 'Yes', then its corollary is whether or not nurses have the right to argue for the reallocation of their care according to a different set of priorities. Nurses, too, it seems could enquire whether caring for, say, five elderly mentally infirm patients equals one coronary artery bypass operation. Asking these questions would put nursing into a much more proactive policy stance than that suggested by the DNE quoted on p. 152. She implied that it was for society to decide what nurses should do – the argument here suggests that nurses could enter the debate themselves. Indeed, if work such as Pearson's (1987) ultimately demonstrates the benefits of nurses having independent skills, then a further corollary is for them to initiate with doctors joint interdisciplinary research into just these areas of concern.

Comparative international data also indicate that the economic marginalization of nursing in the past means using indirect statistics today in order to ask questions about the effective use of nursing care.

Nurses may have shot to the top of the contemporary policy agenda but the lack of meaningful data on their activities has resulted in Parliament, general managers, finance and personnel

directors asking deeply embarrassing questions about the justification for their current deployment.

Table 8.1 shows a set of indicators of health care input and
outcome which compare selected Organization for Economic
Cooperation and Development (OECD) countries on a number of
parameters. The first point to note is that they tell us nothing
meaningful about the relationship between inputs of either medical
or nursing care and standard outcome measures. Indeed, it is
striking that the data are equally bizarre for doctors as for nurses.
Nevertheless, it is the very anomalies which demonstrate how
much more precise such indicators have to be. For example,
column 1 shows two indicators of health care expenditure. First,
purchasing power parity rates in USA dollars per head of population, a standardized measure eliminating the effects of inflation
on individual currencies; second, in parentheses, the percentage of
gross domestic product (GDP – a country's total wealth creation)
devoted to health care. The two figures are not comparable.
Canada and Germany, for example, both spent 8.2% of GDP on
health care in 1982. Yet, in dollars per head of population,
Germany spent just over 80% or four-fifths of the amount spent in
Canada. Further, the differences between the two extremes of the
range show that in Portugal just under half the proportion of its
GDP, 5.7%, was spent on health care compared to the USA's
10.8%. However, in dollars per head of population it is less than
one-fifth of the USA's expenditure. Yet, (Column 4) in terms of
crude mortality, as a measure of outcome, Portugal has a lower
rate than four of the countries which spend more on health care.

What, if anything, can these figures impart about the
relationship of inputs and outcomes in different systems of health
care? If the numbers of physicians and nurses per 10 000 population are considered, the picture becomes even more confused.
Portugal has more doctors than the USA, but less than half as
many as nurses. Australia, with almost the lowest crude mortality
rate has one of the lowest ratios of doctors, and highest of nurses.
Before the beneficial influence of nurses is claimed, however, take
a look at Sweden's figures!

A deeper search of the OECD data throws up, unsurprisingly,
no indicators for the outcomes of nursing care. It does reveal,
however, a wide but unexplained variation between countries for a
range of medical interventions and their outcomes. Clearly the

Table 8.1 Selected indicators for health care expenditure, manpower and health status for selected OECD countries

Selected OECD countries	Per capita expenditure on medical care. Measured at current GDP purchasing power (US $ 1982) health expenditure as % of GDP, 1982, in parentheses[a]	Physicians (per 10000 population, 1980)[b, c]	Nurses (per 10000 population, 1980)[b, c]	Crude mortality rate (per 1000 residential population, 1983[a]
USA	1 388 (10.8)	18.2	51.1	8.5
Sweden	1 239 (9.6)	22.0	88.2	10.9
Canada	1 058 (8.2)*	18.2	N/A	7.0
Germany	883 (8.2)	22.6	54.3	11.7
Australia	796 (7.5)	17.9	82.0	7.1
Italy	607 (7.4)	29.0	N/A	9.9
United Kingdom	539 (6.2)	16.0	39.2	11.7
Portugal	248 (5.7)*	21.1†	22.9†	9.4*

*1982 figures.
†1981 figures.
Sources: a. OECD (1985) Tables 1, 2 and F14.
b. Maxwell (1984).
c. World Health Organization (1984) *Digest of Health Statistics in the European Region of WHO*. WHO Regional Office for Europe.

need for more precise measures of input and outcome becomes increasingly urgent as world-wide debates about the increasing costs of health care become acute. At the end of the day, however, the distribution of available resources is based more on the power to influence governments than through value judgements and moral arguments (Ham, 1981). The earlier hypothetical example of five elderly patients equalling one coronary artery bypass operation will, in the real world, probably be weighted to the right hand side of the equation, and the subsequent effect on nursing is that the pressure for more technically qualified staff is likely to increase. It is notably the shortage of nurses with the technical skills associated with various forms of intensive care which attracts the media attention. Yet Professor Brian Jennett, speaking at the RCN Conference 'In pursuit of excellence in nursing care' (November 1987), claimed that inappropriate care, that which is unnecessary, unsuccessful, unsafe, unkind or unwise, is quite common. He asserted that 10% of medical interventions do more harm than good, and 10% have only a slight benefit. 'Marginal costs', he claimed, 'cannot be afforded'. Although Jennett may be criticized for these unsubstantiated Illich-like (1984) assertions, it may be questioned how marginal are nurses within these marginal costs?

It would neither be desirable nor possible to halt medical innovations. Maxwell (1984), for example, has claimed that there is virtually no limit to the amount that could be spent on health care, pointing out 'although the law of diminishing returns applies, . . . even when the return is small, it may be desperately sought on behalf of the individuals affected'. More searching questions need to be asked, therefore, about the proportionate distribution of resources, especially scarce nursing resources, to what is essentially medical research and development activity. The heart transplant programme, for example, is subject to stringent economic evaluation, about which Buxton (1987) claims that we should not be prepared as a society:

> . . . to devote significant sums of health service resources to programmes that have not been evaluated, however strong their appeal to the public when presented emotionally and dramatically in the media. It is the harsh reality that resources used for one technology in health care cannot be devoted to another.

The opportunity cost of saving one life, or improving its quality, may be the inability to save or improve, two elsewhere.

The current media emphasis on the NHS crisis is confined almost entirely to the acute sector. This lends increasing pressure for a technical hierarchy of nursing skills. The inevitable consequence is for the old, the mentally ill and the socially useless referred to by the DGM at the beginning of this chapter to be cared for by the less skilled, and the unpaid carers discussed above. Is this appropriate, equitable and just? Unless qualified, waged nurses take these issues on board and develop a solidarity with all carers they may end up delegating a large part of the responsibility for the quality of life to the less skilled and the unpaid in our society. This does not mean, of course, that highly qualified nurses should expect to provide all nursing care. Instead, it poses the challenge that the less skilled and the lay carers should not be left behind as the professional drawbridge is pulled up. They too should be considered in debates about overall strategies for care, education, training and remunerative needs.

The invisibility of nursing statistics which has been described results in nurses having difficulty in finding a place in these debates. Yet such evidence as is available shows that nurses are losing ground to doctors in relative increases in staffing. Figure 8.1 shows the accelerating increase in whole time equivalent medical and dental staff compared with a stabilizing situation for nurses between 1983 and 1985 (OHE, 1987a). Do figures such as these demonstrate that the present health care crisis is, at least in part, fuelled by supplier-led medical demand? If so, given that overall in-patient lengths of stay have decreased by 33% since 1965 and that discharges and deaths per available bed have increased by 50% since 1970 (OHE, 1987b, c), perhaps it is not surprising that nursing wastage rates give rise to such concern. But what too is the impact on the unpaid carers who invisibly share the burden of this increased productivity and hospital efficiency?

Importantly from the patient's point of view, is the question how effectively and efficiently are the nurses who remain deployed? Answers will always be fraught with ethical and moral issues, but at present without the information, it is difficult for nurses even to enter the debate.

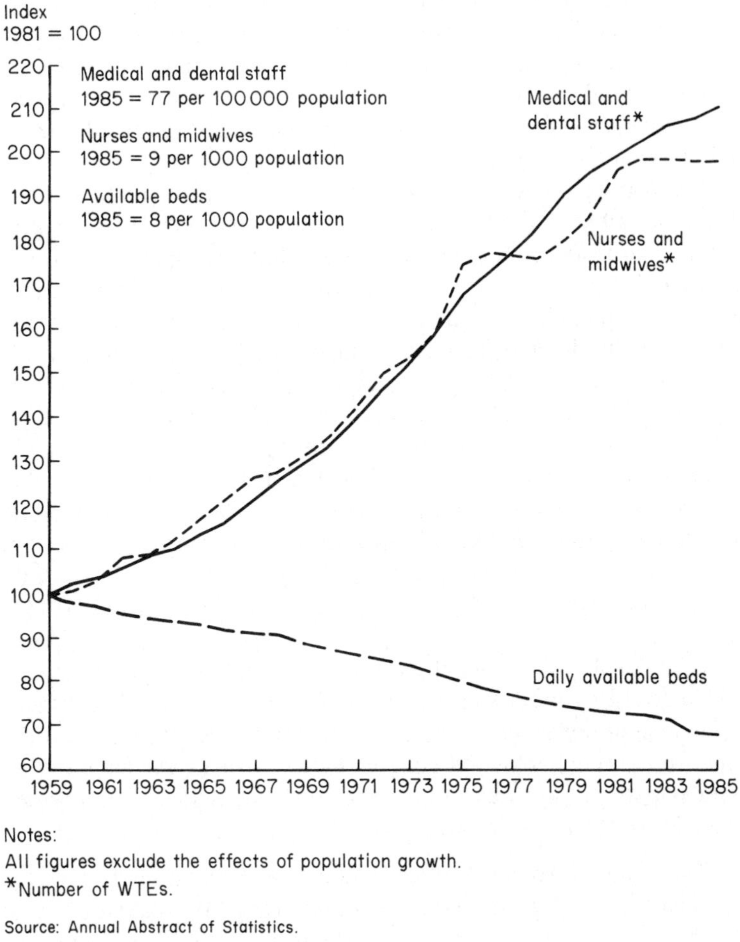
Index
1981 = 100
220
210
200
190
180
170
160
150
140
130
120
110
100
90
80
70
60
Medical and dental staff
1985 = 77 per 100 000 population
Nurses and midwives
1985 = 9 per 1000 population
Available beds
1985 = 8 per 1000 population
Medical and
dental staff*
Nurses and
midwives*
Daily available beds
1959 1961 1963 1965 1967 1969 1971 1973 1975 1977 1979 1981 1983 1985
Notes:
All figures exclude the effects of population growth.
*Number of WTEs.
Source: Annual Abstract of Statistics.

Figure 8.1 NHS hospital available beds, medical and dental staff, and nurses and midwives.

SOME CONCLUDING THOUGHTS

Nursing as caring, and caring as a women's issue are currently both marginalized policy issues. Reverby (1987) cited at the beginning of this chapter (p. 152), claimed that contemporary nursing's central dilemma is the order to care in a society which refuses to value caring. This, in a nutshell, is the major present cause for concern. In this chapter, an attempt has been made to set out a related agenda which nurses could address. There are, however, some further issues relating to the gendered division of caring labour which also need to be carried forward.

It has been argued that the marginalization of caring occurs in both the public and domestic domains, and that policies for waged nursing are subordinate to the overriding dominant claims of medicine, especially in the acute sector. The absence of much hard data to support this argument is, in policy terms, predictable. Data are normally defined, collected and debated in order to advance the understanding of major policy concerns. Neither nursing nor caring have, until recently, demanded much attention in terms of labour force statistics. Changes in current policy could easily result in expedient solutions. In a political climate which favours the operation of market forces it would be very easy to remunerate more highly those nurses whose shortage hits the daily news. In recognizing the ubiquity of caring as women's work nurses could reflect, however, on what equity in health care really means (RCN, 1987).

If the subordination of caring as women's work is to be challenged then nurses as women will also have to challenge their own assumptions about caring being their sole prerogative. To open up caring across the gender divide involves challenging the sexual bias of skill definition which Phillips and Taylor (1980) describe in the following way:

> The work of women is often deemed inferior simply because it is women who do it. Women workers carry into the workplace their status as subordinate individuals, and this status comes to define the value of the work they do. Far from being an objective economic fact, skill is often an ideological category imposed on certain types of work by virtue of the sex and power of the workers who perform it.

However much women may complain about this state of affairs there is also a paradoxical sense of security in hiding behind it as a justification for the continuing experience of oppression. The relentless continuation of this paradox can be seen in nurses' ambivalence over the domination of senior health care and nursing posts by men, whilst at the same time the evidence suggests that they are often reluctant to come forward for consideration for such jobs themselves. Despite the evidence of 'a climate hostile to women' (Davies and Rosser, 1986) there has been little use of tribunals by nurses to challenge the process of sexual discrimination in the upper echelons of the NHS.

At the other end of the spectrum, there is considerable ambivalence amongst women in general about the taking over by men of some of the traditional caring functions. Yet Arbor and Gilbert (in press) found in a study of the elderly disabled that of those living with someone else (two-thirds of the total) over one-third of the carers were men. Of these carers, three-quarters were spouses or unmarried sons. Furthermore, an exactly equal number of caring spouses were male and female.

The avant-garde model in community care is San Francisco's gay men buddies in AIDS, but this also offers an unspoken legitimation for a caring model for all gay men. Why should this not be a model for all men? Historical precedent rather than empirical evidence may suggest not, but in view of the problem of AIDS world wide, the change in the supply and demand for women's labour, and the continuing pool of unemployed men, then the time may be ripe for change in our assumptions and our attitudes.

Achieving a fair and just distribution of resources is fraught with both economic and moral difficulties in any system of caring (Mooney and McGuire, 1987). Nevertheless, if waged nurses could pause momentarily to reflect on the wider policy implications of the marginalization of caring as women's work, then they might find cause for increased mutual solidarity. This solidarity would, however, require a challenge to the many preconceptions about women and work. It would demand, first, the recognition that caring is labour wherever it is carried out and therefore requires partnership across the sectors, and appropriate rewards. Second, it needs a paradigm shift in order for our gendered assumptions about the division of caring labour to be broken down. These two conditions may seem difficult to achieve, but together they offer the possibility of hope rather than concern for the future. If waged nurses could begin to reflect on the issues, then they might be better prepared to initiate some of the challenges which they contain.

NOTES

1. Feminist authors have not, of course, completely ignored waged nursing care. Oakley (1984), Salvage (1985) and Davies and Rosser (1986) are important contributors to this field. Nevertheless, because of the nature of their respective briefs, they have concentrated on the waged sector to the exclusion of nursing as caring in a general sense.

2. Before problems can find a place on the policy agenda they have to be defined in terms which are relevant to the interests of powerful proponents of the issues. Routinely collected social statistics are not, therefore, neutral artefacts but have life histories which are socially constructed. Even such apparently neutral statistics as infant and perinatal mortality have been defined in terms which have changed over time, and which have been used in order to serve particular policy ends (Armstrong, 1986; Robinson 1986).

REFERENCES

Adam, S. (1987) Women do the work but men get the status (book review) *Health Service Journal*, **97**, 26 Nov, 1389.

Armstrong, D. (1986) The invention of infant mortality. *Sociology of Health and Illness*, **8**(3) Sep, 211–32.

Bachrach, P. and Baratz, M.S. (1962) The two faces of power. *American Political Science Review*, **56**, 947–52.

Baldwin, S. and Glendinning, C. (1983) Employment, women and their disabled children, in *A Labour of Love: Women, Work and Caring*, (eds J. Finch, and D. Groves), Routledge and Kegan Paul, London.

Brown, C.A. (1975) Women workers in the health service industry. *International Journal of Health Services*, **5**(2), 173–84.

Bullough, B. (1975) Barriers to the nurse practitioner movement: problems of women in a woman's field. *International Journal of Health Services*, **5**(2), 225–33.

Buxton, M. (1987) The economic evaluation of high technology medicine: the case of heart transplants, in *Health and Economics* (ed A. Williams), Macmillan, London.

Carpenter, M. (1978) Managerialism and the division of labour in nursing, in *Readings in the Sociology of Nursing*. (eds R. Dingwall and J. McIntosh), Churchill Livingstone, Edinburgh.

Carpenter, M. (1980) Asylum nursing before 1914: a chapter in the history of labour, in *Re-writing Nursing History*, (ed. C. Davies), Croom Helm, London.

Clay, T. (1987) *Nurses, Power and Politics*. Heinemann, London.

Davies, C. and Rosser, J. (1986) *Processes of Discrimination: Report on a Study of Women Working in the NHS*, Department of Health and Social Security, London.

Dean, M. and Boulton, G. (1980) The administration of poverty and the development of nursing practice in nineteenth-century England, in *Rewriting Nursing History* (ed. C. Davies), Croom Helm, London.

Delamothe, T. (1988) Nursing grievances 1: voting with their feet. *British Medical Journal*, **296**, 2 Jan, 25–8.

Dingwall, R., Eekelaar, J. and Murray, T. (1983) *The Protection of Children: State Intervention and Family Life.* Blackwell, Oxford.

Donnison, J. (1977) *Midwives and Medical Men: a History of Interprofessional Rivalries and Women's rights.* Heinemann, London.

Evans, J. (1986) Feminism within the discipline of political science: feminist theory and political analysis, in *Feminism and political theory* (ed. J. Evans), Sage, London.

Finch, J. (1984) Community care: developing non-sexist alternatives. *Critical Social Policy*, **9** Spring, 6–18.

Finch, J. and Groves, D. (eds) (1983) *A Labour of Love: Women, Work and Caring.* Routledge and Kegan Paul, London.

Gamarnikow, E. (1978) Sexual divisions of labour: the case of nursing, in *Feminism and Materialism: Women and Modes of Production* (eds A. Kuhn and A.-M. Wolpe), Routledge and Kegan Paul, London.

Graham, H. (1979) Prevention and health: every mother's business: a comment on child health policies in the 70s in *The Sociology of the Family: New Directions for Britain* (ed. C. Harris), University of Keele, Keele (Sociological review monograph 28).

Graham, H. (1985) Providers, negotiators and mediators: women as the hidden carers, in *Women, Health and Healing: Toward a New Perspective* (eds E. Lewin and V. Elesen), Tavistock, London.

Gray, A.M. (1987) *The Economics of Nursing: a Review of the Literature Review.* Nursing Policy Studies Centre, University of Warwick, Coventry (Nursing policy studies 2).

Groves, D. and Finch, J. (1983) Natural selection: perspectives on entitlement to the invalid care allowance, in *A Labour of Love: Women, Work and Caring* (eds J. Finch and D. Groves), Routledge and Kegan Paul, London.

Ham, C. (1981) *Policy-making in the National Health Service.* Macmillan, London.

Henderson, V. (1966) *The Nature of Nursing.* Macmillan, New York.

Jennett, B. (1984) *High Technology Medicine; Benefits and Burdens.* Nuffield Provincial Hospitals Trust, London (Rock Carling Fellowship 1983).

Jennett, B. (1987) *Quality – a Medical View.* Unpublished paper given at the Royal College of Nursing Conference, In pursuit of excellence, held in London 2–4 November.

Kalisch, B. and Kalisch, P. (1985) Nurses on strike: labour management conflict in U.S. hospitals in the role of the press, *Political Issues in Nursing: Past, Present and Future*, vol. 1, (ed. R. White) Wiley, Chichester.

Kitson, A.L. (1987) A comparative analysis of lay-caring and professional (nursing) care relationships. *International Journal of Nursing Studies*, **24**(2), 155–65.

Land, H. (1982) The family wage, *The Woman Question: Readings in the Subordination of Women* (ed. M. Evans), Fontana, Oxford.

Leininger, M. (1981) *Care: An Essential Human Need*. Slack, Thorofare.

Leininger, M. (1984) *Care: The Essence of Nursing and Health*. Slack, Thorofare.

Lewin, E. (1977) Feminist ideology and the meaning of work. *Catalyst*, (10/11), 78–103.

Lukes, S. (1986) *Power: A Radical View*. Macmillan, London.

Maggs, C.J. (1983) *The Origins of General Nursing*. Croom Helm, London.

Maxwell, R.J. (1984) International comparisons: what can we learn? in *Health Care UK: an Economic, Social and Policy Audit* (eds A. Harrison and J. Gretton), Chartered Institute of Public Finance and Accountancy, London.

Maynard, A. (1987) Markets and health care, in *Health and Economics* (ed. A. Williams), Macmillan, London.

Melosh, B. (1986) Nursing and Reagonomics: cost containment in the United States, in *Political Issues in Nursing: Past, Present and Future*, Vol 2. (ed. R. White), Wiley, Chichester.

Milio, N. (1985) Nursing within the ecology of public policy: a case in point, in *Political Issues in Nursing: Past, Present and Future*, Vol. 1. (ed. R. White), Wiley, Chichester.

Mooney, G. and McGuire, A. (1987) Distributive justice with special reference to geographical inequality in health care, in *Health and Economics* (ed. A. Williams), Macmillan, London.

National Audit Office (1985) *Report by the Comptroller and Auditor General: National Health Service: control of nursing manpower*. HMSO, London.

NHS Management Inquiry Team (1983) *NHS Management Inquiry: (letter to the Secretary of State)* The Team, London (Team leader E.R. Griffiths).

Oakley, A. (1984) *The Captured Womb: A History of the Pregnant Women*. Blackwell, Oxford.

Office of Health Economics (1987a) NHS hospital available beds, medical and dental staff, and nurses and midwives, UK, in *Compendium of Health Statistics*, 6th edn, OHE, London, Figure 3.10.

Office of Health Economics (1987b) NHS hospital inpatients average length of stay, England, in *Compendium of Health Statistics*, 6th edn, OHE, London, Table 3.31.

Office of Health Economics (1987c) NHS hospital inpatients: discharges and deaths per available bed by speciality, England, in *Compendium of Health Statistics*, 6th edn, OHE, London, Table 3.28. 43.

Olesen, V. and Lewin, E. (1985) Women, health and healing: a theoretical introduction, in *Women, Health and Healing: Toward a New Perspective* (eds E. Lewin and V. Olesen), Tavistock, London.

Organisation for Economic Cooperation and Development (1985) *Measuring Health Care 1960–1983: Expenditure, Costs and Performance.* OECD, Paris (Social policy studies 2).

Pascall, G. (1986) *Social Policy: a Feminist Analysis.* Tavistock, London.

Pearson, A. (ed.) (1987) *Primary Nursing: Nursing in the Burford and Oxford Nursing Development Units.* Croom Helm, London.

Phillips, A. (1987) Neglect that forces nurses off the wards. *Independent,* 16 Nov, 16.

Phillips, A., and Taylor, B. (1980) Sex and skill: notes towards a feminist economics, *Feminist Review,* **6**, 79–88.

Pizurki, H., Mejia, A., Butter, I. and Ewart, L. (eds) (1987) *Women as Providers of Health Care.* World Health Organization, Geneva.

Reverby, S.M. (1987) *Ordered to Care: the Dilemma of American Nursing, 1850–1945.* Cambridge University Press, Cambridge.

Rimmer, L. (1983) The economics of work and caring, in *A Labour of love: women, work and caring* (eds J. Finch and D. Groves), Routledge and Kegan Paul, London.

Robinson, J. (1982) *An Evaluation of Health Visiting.* Council for the Education and Training of Health Visitors, London.

Robinson, J.J.A. (1986) *A study of the policy implications arising from a local survey of perinatal mortality.* Unpublished PhD thesis, University of Keele.

Robinson, J. and Strong, P. (1987) *Professional nursing advice after Griffiths: an interim report.* Nursing Policy Studies Centre, University of Warwick, Coventry (Nursing policy studies 1).

Royal College of Nursing (1987) *In Pursuit of Excellence: A Position Statement on Nursing.* RCN, London

Salvage, J. (1985) *The Politics of Nursing.* Heinemann, London.

Schulman, S. (1958) Basic functional roles in nursing: mother surrogate and healer, in *Patients, Physicians and Illness* (ed. E. Gartly Jaco), Free Press, New York.

Schulman, S. (1972) Mother surrogate – after a decade, in *Patients, Physicians and Illness* (ed. E. Gartly Jaco), 2nd edn, Free Press, New York.

Review Body for Nursing Staff, Midwives, Health Visitors and Professions Allied to Medicine (1987) *Fourth Report on Nursing Staff, Midwives and Health Visitors.* HMSO, London.

Secretariat for Futures Studies (1984) *Time to Care: a Report Prepared for the Swedish Secretariat for Futures Studies.* Pergamon, Oxford.

Smith, D. (1974) Women's perspective as a radical critique of sociology. *Sociological Inquiry,* **44**(1), 7–13.

Smith, F.B. (1982) *Florence Nightingale: Reputation and Power.* Croom Helm, London.

Stacey, M. (1981) The division of labour revisited, or, overcoming the two Adams, in *Practice and Progress: British Sociology 1950–1980* (eds P. Abrams,, R. Deem, J. Finch and P. Rock), Allen and Unwin, London.

Stacey, M. (1987) *Gender and the Division of Health Labour: Past and*

Present. Presidential address to the Society for the Social History of Medicine, 4 December. Department of Sociology, University of Warwick, Coventry.

Strong, P.M. and Robinson, J.A. (1988) *New Model Management: Griffiths and the NHS.* Nursing Policy Studies Centre, University of Warwick, Coventry (in prep.).

Ungerson, C. (1983) Why do women care? in *A Labour of Love: Women, Work and Caring* (eds J. Finch and D. Groves), Routledge and Kegan Paul, London.

Ungerson, C. (1987) *Policy is Personal: Sex, Gender, and Informal Care.* Tavistock, London.

Walker, A. (1983) Care for elderly people: a conflict between women and the state, in *A Labour of Love: Women, Work and Caring* (eds J. Finch and D. Groves), Routledge and Kegan Paul, London.

White, R. (1978) *Social Change and the Development of the Nursing Profession: a Study of the Poor Law Nursing Service 1848–1948.* Kimpton, London.

Whittaker, E. and Olesen, V. (1964) The faces of Florence Nightingale: functions of the heroine legend in an occupational sub-culture. *Human Organization,* **23**(2) Summer, 123–30.

Williams, A. (ed.) (1987a) *Health and Economics.* Macmillan, London.

Williams, A. (1987b) Health economics: the cheerful face of the dismal service, in *Health and Economics* (ed. A. Williams) Macmillan, London.

Wilson, V. (1971) An analysis of femininity in nursing. *American Behavioural Scientist,* **15**(2) 213–20.

Index